Asian Voices

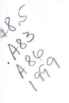

Asian Voices

Asian and Asian American Health Educators Speak Out

Edited by

Lin Zhan, PhD, RN

Faculty, University of Massachusetts
Research Fellow, Institute of Asian American Studies
Boston, Massachusetts

JONES AND BARTLETT PUBLISHERS
Sudbury, Massachusetts
BOSTON   TORONTO   LONDON   SINGAPORE

World Headquarters
Jones and Bartlett Publishers
40 Tall Pine Drive
Sudbury, MA 01776
978-443-5000
800-832-0034
info@jbpub.com
www.jbpub.com

Jones and Bartlett Publishers Canada
P.O. Box 19020
Toronto, ON M5S 1X1
CANADA

Jones and Bartlett Publishers International
Barb House, Barb Mews
London W6 7PA
UK

> The views expressed in this publication represent the views of the authors and do not necessarily reflect the official views of the National League for Nursing.

Library of Congress Cataloging-in-Publication Data

Asian voices : Asian and Asian American health educators speak out /
    edited by Lin Zhan.
        p.   cm.
    Includes bibliographical references and index.
    ISBN 0-7637-0922-0
    1. Asian Americans—Medical care.   2. Asians—Medical care.
3. Asian Americans—Health and hygiene.   4. Asians—Health and
hygiene.   5. Transcultural medical care.   I. Zhan, Lin.
II. National League for Nursing.
[DNLM: 1. Asian Americans.   2. Public Health—United States.
3. Health Promotion—United States.   4. Health Education—United
States.   5. Education, Nursing.   WA 300 A832 1998]
RA448.5.A83A86   1998
362.1' 089' 95073—DC21
DNLM/DLC
for Library of Congress   97-34603
                                                              CIP

Printed in the United States of America
02 01 00 99 98   10 9 8 7 6 5 4 3 2 1

To our colleagues—faculty, students, clinicians, and community men and women—who helped us create a better vision of healthcare for all. Nothing is more rewarding than to work with this book's authors, who humbled me immediately.

To my parents, Da Fong Zahn and Hui Jue He, who were my first teachers and always inspire me to care about others. To Min Xiao, who provided patience and support throughout this production.

Contributing Authors

Anli Jiang, MED
Associate Professor
Chief Secretary of Nursing
Director, Department of Basic
    Nursing
Nursing Department, Second Military
    Medical University
Shanghai, Peoples Republic of China

Clementina D. Ceria, PhD, RN
Assistant Professor
School of Nursing
University of Hawaii at Manoa
Honolulu, Hawaii

Connie S. Chan, PhD
Co-Director, Institute of Asian
    American Studies
University of Massachusetts
Boston, Massachusetts

Sandra E. Gibson, EdD, ARNP
Associate Professor
School of Nursing
Barry University
Miami Shores, Florida

Zibin Guo, PhD
Department of Social Medicine
Harvard Medical School
Boston, Massachusetts

Jillian Inouye, PhD, RN
Associate Professor and Coordinator
Graduate Community Mental Health
    Nursing Program
School of Nursing
University of Hawaii at Manoa
Honolulu, Hawaii

Dianne N. Ishida, PhD, RN
Associate Professor
School of Nursing
University of Hawaii at Manoa
Honolulu, Hawaii

Ide Pang Katims, PhD, RN
Assistant Professor and Director
Department of Nursing
The State University of New York
New Paltz, New York

Yi Chun Lo, MA, RN
Associate Director,
Center for Career Advancement
National League for Nursing
New York, New York

Kem B. Louie, PhD, RN, CS, FAAN
Professor and Chairperson
Graduate Nursing Programs
College of Mount Saint Vincent
Bronx, New York

Michiyo Mizuno, PHN, MSN, RN
Assistant Professor
The School of Health Sciences
Tokai University
Bohseidai, Isehara-shi
Kanagawa, (259-11), Japan

A. Gigi V. Moneda, MSN, ARNP
Adjunct Faculty
Florida International University
    School of Nursing
North Miami Beach, Florida
Miami Shores, Florida

Kyung Rim Shin, EdD, RN
Associate Dean
Department of Nursing
EHWA Woman's University
Seodeamun-Ku
Seoul, Korea

Yoshiko Shimamoto, PhD, RN
School of Nursing
University of Hawaii at Manoa
Honolulu, Hawaii

Shu-Zhen Li, MD
Nursing Department
Second Military Medical University
Shanghai, Peoples Republic of China

Geraldine Valencia-Go, PhD, RN, CS
Associate Professor of Nursing
Chairperson, Undergraduate Programs
    in Nursing
School of Nursing
College of New Rochelle
New Rochelle, New York

Paul Y. Watanabe, PhD
Co-Director, Institute of Asian
    American Studies
University of Massachusetts
Boston, Massachusetts

Lin Zhan, PhD, RN
Assistant Professor
College of Nursing
Research Fellow
Institute of Asian American
    Studies
University of Massachusetts
Boston, Massachusetts
and Director, Educational Councils
National League for Nursing
New York, New York

Foreword

Americans from Asia have resided in the United States for well over 150 years. Currently, over 10 million Americans trace their ancestry to Asia. By the middle of the twenty-first century, the U.S. Census Bureau estimates that over 10% of the U.S. population will be of Asian descent.

Despite their long history in the United States and their impressive numbers, Asian Americans have remained relatively invisible in this land where they have settled and reared families. History books and school curricula give short shrift to their experience. In political and policymaking circles, Asian Americans have struggled for a seat at the table. In the words of historian Ronald Takaki, Asian Americans, for the most part, have been regarded as "strangers from a different shore."

In the health field as well, knowledge about and contributions by Asian Americans have not been accorded proper recognition. This is an especially critical failing. Health issues left inadequately addressed have consequences that extend well beyond the individuals directly affected—to their families and communities, and even to the larger society in which they dwell.

Healthcare educators, therefore, face the vital challenge of shedding light into a realm where relative darkness exists. This volume represents a significant effort to respond to this challenge. In these chapters, healthcare issues facing Asian and Asian American communities are explored, useful insights on health promotion and nursing education are shared, and the goals of high quality and culturally competent care are substantially advanced.

Just as important as the topics discussed in this book are the individuals assembled to address them. Often in the past, Asian American voices have been ignored or silenced, contributing to neglect and invisibility. Fortunately in these pages, Asian and Asian American health educator

voices *are* heard. This in itself is a notable achievement. These contributors will assuredly educate us all, and their willingness to speak should inspire others to do the same.

PAUL Y. WATANABE, PhD AND CONNIE S. CHAN, PhD
Co-Directors
Institute for Asian American Studies
University of Massachusetts Boston

Preface

Asian Voices: Asian and Asian American Health Educators Speak Out is the third book in the NLN Press series dedicated to exploring health concerns of various culture groups. For the first time in history, the National League for Nursing has reached out to Asian and Asian American educators who, while making significant contributions to healthcare and education, have remained relatively invisible. Asian Americans now are the fastest growing ethnic minority in the United States. Their population is expected to increase from the current 3% to more than 10% by 2030. Yet, a paucity of literature and research data exists concerning health education and healthcare of Asian communities, especially in the nursing literature. Timely, this book addresses critical health and health related issues facing Asian communities.

When I was first approached about writing this book by NLN Press Director Allan Graubard, I was thrilled. Immediately I asked myself, "What messages should we convey to readers in advancing our understandings of health and healthcare for Asian Americans?" I sent out the "call for manuscripts" to invite "voices" from Asian and Asian American health educators. Overwhelming responses were received. The development and conceptualization of this book involved many decisions, including selection of content and authors. Content selection was open-ended with little structure and guidance, which allowed authors the freedom to express their opinions, share research outcomes with readers, and voice concerns on the healthcare of Asians and Asian American Pacific Islanders (AAPIs). Voices included in this book come from four predominant Asian subgroups: Chinese, Korean, Japanese, and Filipino, and from eight geographical areas: China, Japan, Korea, Florida, Hawaii, Massachusetts, New Jersey, and New York. Contributors to this book are known locally, regionally, and internationally. Book production involved the efforts and support of many individuals. Allan Graubard and Nancy Jeffries, NLN Press senior editor, were instrumental in reviewing and organizing this book. Many of my colleagues, Asians and Americans alike, offered ongoing support and encouragement. Specifically, I want to thank all the contributors who shared their voices and made this book a reality.

What emerged in this book were some major issues facing healthcare educators, researchers, and practitioners who work with and provide care for Asians: lack of reliable and valid data in relation to health of Asian Americans; inaccessible healthcare services; conflict in health belief models and practices; and the myth of Asian Americans as "model minority," perpetuating the false notion that this population consists, for the most part, of healthy people who need minimal health related research and services. Voices as such were echoed in the document *Healthy People 2,000* (U.S. Department of Health and Human Services, 1992). As you read this book, you will hear the voices of Asian and Asian American health educators as they share their diverse cultures, knowledge, experience, research, and insights related to healthcare issues in Asian communities.

CONTENT OVERVIEW

This book is organized into thirteen chapters with three major themes: health promotion and disease prevention, healthcare and health related issues, and nursing education. Part I consists of three chapters. Chapter 1 offers an overview of major health problems experienced by AAPIs, which include, but are not limited to, cerebrovascular disease, cancer, chronic hepatitis B, smoking, HIV/AIDS, and mental illness. The author suggests strategies to reduce health risk factors among AAPIs. Chapter 2 describes experiences of a group of older Filipino women who, like many other immigrants, came to the United States experiencing feelings of loneliness, displacement, social isolation, cultural conflict, and lack of access to the mainstream healthcare system. Instead of dwelling in despair, this group of older Filipino women proactively formed the "Health Promotion Program for Golden Dreamers." Helped by Filipino nurses and nurse practitioners, dreams were realized and the health promotion program became a cultural center where health related issues and concerns were discussed, cultural education took place, and the expression of cultural pride was evident. Chapter 3 discusses health practices for older Chinese American women. The Chinese view of aging, *Xi Young Hong,* a bright red color at sunset (an analogy to aging) and traditional health beliefs play important roles in health promotion and disease prevention, as was exemplified by *yin* and *yang*—the notion representing two opposite forces dialectically related to one another. Yet language difficulties, financial barriers, and cultural and healthcare conflicts impede older Chinese American women in obtaining proper healthcare. Even more startling, the image of Asians as immigrant role models has disguised the enduring poverty of some. Authors call for culturally sensitive and appropriate health programs to reduce health disparities in AAPIs. They also remind readers that cautions must be made when lumping together AAPIs in designing health programs, because this group is not homogeneous; it is composed of over 60 ethnic groups, 40 different languages, from more than 20 countries.

Part II consists of seven chapters that explore healthcare issues in the United States and other countries. Chapter 4 advances our knowledge of Korean women's health, historically delayed because of social prejudices against women and the vagaries of industrialization, which centered more on economic development than women's health. Such negligence has resulted in an increased mortality rate among Korean women caused by cancer, AIDS, and suicide. The author suggests a community-based approach to improve women's rights and their involvement in decision making in relation to their health. This chapter helps health professionals understand unique health problems facing Korean women and the social context that contributed to these problems.

Chapter 5, based on a qualitative study, offers cultural insights with respect to how some Filipino widows successfully coped with their grief. They reconstructed their lives, acquired new roles, and eventually gained independence. Equally significant, they were liberated from a traditional culture by which widows' children were considered as properties of their in-laws and worse; widows could not remarry freely and suffered abuse and humiliation from in-laws and society. This chapter guides health professionals to identify coping strategies for grieving Filipino widows. General health problems in Filipino Americans are discussed in Chapter 6, including a high percentage of low birth weight babies (10 per 100 Filipino births) and lack of prenatal care and immunization in the first 24 months of life. Readers are presented with Filipino culture: *Amor propio* (sense of self-esteem and self-worth), *Hiya* (self-depreciation and shame), *Pakikisama* (a means of enforcing smooth interpersonal relationships), and *Bahala Na* (leaving things to fate or God). How culture as such influences Filipinos' thinking and health-seeking behaviors is discussed. Future research agendas for the health of Filipino Americans are suggested.

Chapter 7 explores HIV/AIDS issues in Asian Americans. These issues have been neglected due to a lack of incidence reports and reliable data at local and national levels. Authors critique that campaigns against HIV/AIDS have largely centered on the North American culture. This approach is ineffective to the AAPI population because many of the AAPI immigrants are not only monolingual, but also illiterate in their own language. Communication difficulties result in a lack of understanding the multifaceted HIV/AIDS issues. Authors suggest using multilingual information, selecting appropriate sites for distribution of HIV/AIDS related information, establishing AAPI community networks, and overcoming cultural barriers to initiate a dialogue on HIV/AIDS.

Buddhism, Taoism, and Confucianism are very much of the traditional Chinese, Japanese, and Southeast Asian way of life. Buddhism, for example, has influenced almost every Asian society for more than two thousand years. How does Buddhism affect decision making with regard to end-of-life issues? This is the very question health professionals raise in daily practice. Chapter 8, titled "Buddhist Ethics and Implications for End-of-Life Issues," opens our eyes to this question and the search for its answers. The moral framework of Buddhism demands a holistic, humanistic, and organic view of life and death. Buddhists believe a person represents a psycho-physical totality of the human being consisting of many lifetimes, including rebirth and Karma after death. Understanding the Buddhist cosmological belief helps health practitioners to avoid imposing their own meanings and beliefs when dealing with end-of-life issues.

Chapter 9 reveals the findings of a triangulation study that examined the dynamics between cultural factors and Chinese Americans' health-seeking behaviors. The author identifies major factors affecting Chinese immigrants' health seeking behaviors and decisions that include, but are not limited to, language barriers, lack of knowledge about American society and its healthcare system, different cultural assumptions about health and illness, stereotypes, intergenerational conflict, and discrimination. One informant in this study, for example, provided a vivid description: "American healthcare system is like another puzzle that exists in a puzzling society." Chapter 10 introduces readers to a very different Japanese healthcare system, challenged by a rapidly increasing elderly population. The author presents changes and strategies adopted by public health services and the medical society in Japan. Japanese cultural characteristics, the role of Japanese nursing, and how these factors affect the delivery of healthcare are discussed.

Frequently, health educators ask how ethnic minority students learn in an American classroom. Faculty expect students to participate, display individualism, and ask questions in their learning. However, other cultures may have far different norms. Does learning to learn serve as a bridge between cultures? Part III of this book offers readers understanding in this area. Chapter 11 discusses the use of a culturally appropriate tutorial approach—problem-based learning. This tutorial method created an environment in which Asian students felt comfortable to participate and voice their opinions, transforming the traditional role of the tutor as a main source of knowledge and wisdom to students who took ownership in learning. Chapter 12 surveys the historical development of higher education for nurses in Taiwan, or the Republic of China. Exemplar cases of Taiwanese nurses in the United States are presented. The author suggests competencies to meet the demands and challenges of the changing healthcare environment in Taiwan.

As more Americans seek non-Western medicine, questions such as "What is Chinese medicine?" are raised. Chapter 13, written by experienced clinicians, offers a detailed explanation of traditional Chinese medicine and its theoretical propositions and interventions. Techniques of acupuncture and moxibustion are depicted by more than 15 figures in this chapter. An understanding of Chinese medicine helps health professionals intervene with Asian clients, who very often are treated by Western medicine while following traditional Chinese medicine. This chapter can be used as a reference in understanding the interplay between two very different medical approaches.

IN CLOSING

Voices in this book represent Asian and AAPI health and healthcare issues. This book is by no means a complete picture; it was written, in part, to fill the gap in educational materials on healthcare of Asian communities. It helps readers recognize the diverse cultural dimensions, characteristics, experiences, needs, and barriers in four Asian subgroups: Chinese, Filipino, Japanese, and Korean. Voices in this book call for more health related research and aggregate databases for Asians and AAPIs. Information and knowledge generated from these voices will improve cultural competency for healthcare providers and educators in their work. As the United States becomes ever more diverse, healthcare

providers have a professional responsibility to understand the populations for whom we care and with whom we work. American society
today is really a connection of intertwining cultures, each bringing its
own character and palpable contributions to the nation. How we deal
with this interconnectedness bears significant implications on the quality
of life for all Americans as well as for AAPIs.

LIN ZHAN, PhD, RN
Faculty, University of Massachusetts Boston
Research Fellow, Institute of Asian American Studies
Director, Educational Councils, NLN

Contents

PART I

Health Promotion

CHAPTER ONE

Health Promotion Interventions for Asian American Pacific Islanders

Kem B. Louie, PhD, RN, CS, FAAN

In this era of managed care, with its focus on utilizing cost-effective services, prevention becomes ever more important. Health prevention interventions early in the course of disease or even before disease develops have contributed to substantial reductions in morbidity and mortality rates. For example, age adjusted mortality from strokes has decreased by more than 50% since 1972. This rate has been associated with earlier detection and treatment of hypertension (Casper, Wing, Strogatz, Davis, & Tyroler, 1992). Identified as the most promising role for prevention is changing the personal habits of individuals long before health problems develop. McGinnis and Foege (1993) estimated that nearly half of all deaths occurring in the United States in 1990 were attributed to external factors such as tobacco, alcohol, and illicit drug use; diet and activity; motor vehicle accidents; and sexual behavior.

HEALTH PROMOTION AND ETHNICITY

Cultural factors such as ethnicity play a role in the understanding of health. In the Health Promotion Model developed by Pender (1996), the framework integrated nursing and behavioral science perspectives on factors influencing health behaviors. Demographic factors such as age, gender, race, ethnicity, and education influence personal factors; personal factors include individual perceptions of health, self-esteem, one's definition of health, and perceived benefits of health-promoting behaviors.

In a recent article, Chen (1996) generated a substantive theory that describes and explains beliefs and behaviors of health promotion and ill-

3

ness prevention among Chinese elderly living in the United States. In a grounded study of 21 Tai elderly, the author found that conformity with nature is the fundamental belief in which a person achieves health and wellness. This is the process of knowing nature and trying one's best to modify oneself to fit the laws of nature. Three interrelated subprocesses—harmonizing with the environment, following bliss, and listening to heaven—also were identified in maintaining health.

Frye (1995) reviewed 106 articles and 93 interviews with refugees and professionals in the health promotion field to identify cultural themes related to Vietnamese, Cambodian, and Hmong refugee populations. The purpose was to design culturally appropriate health promotion strategies for these groups. Two cultural themes emerged: kinship solidarity and the search for equilibrium. Various strategies in which health information could be disseminated included recognition of cultural illness, the use of folklore, and cultural knowledge in understanding family structure transitions, depression, and substance abuse.

Caring for clients and families from diverse Asian American Pacific Islander (AAPI) cultures poses further challenges. This population's traditional beliefs of health and illness vary with Western views. Specifically, a majority of AAPI groups believe that health is a balance of forces or energies while Western society defines health as the absence of illness. There are 53 AAPI subgroups, each with its own language, culture, and history of immigration (Lin-Fu, 1993). This chapter examines the incidences and prevalence rates of health problems affecting AAPIs and discusses culture-specific health promotion strategies.

HEALTH PROBLEMS: INCIDENCE AND PREVALENCE RATES

Cardiovascular Disease

Enas (1996) reported that the predominant form of cardiovascular disease (CVD) in Western societies as coronary artery disease (CAD), while in Asian societies cerebrovascular disease, or stroke, is more common. The high stroke rate among Asians is generally attributed to uncontrolled hypertension, which is related to high salt intake. The rate of stroke mortality among AAPIs is similar to that of other groups. Among Asian groups, for example, the Japanese have the lowest CAD rate while Asian Indians have the highest CAD rate of any ethnic group studied. Enas reported that, upon immigration, Asian Americans experience a decreased rate of stroke and an increased rate of CAD, and associated this variation with one's degree of acculturation. Higher rates are attributed to increased intake of cholesterol and animal fat, which results in dyslipidemia, the major risk factor for CAD. Asian Indians have higher levels of lipoprotein, a genetically determined risk factor for premature atherosclerosis, multi-vessel disease, premature stroke, and peripheral vascular disease.

Risk Factors. Risk factors for CVD include hypertension, diabetes, increased cholesterol, decreased physical activity, salt and animal fat in the diet, the act of smoking, and obesity. Health-risk assessments, in all health-care settings, identify one's degree of risk for this disease.

Screening for blood cholesterol and lipoproteins is encouraged for males between 35 and 65 years of age and women between 45 and 65. Genetic counseling for familial lipoproteins is particularly important for East Indians.

Teaching on CVD requires an understanding of the disease process and nutritional factors that lower one's risk, such as decreasing intake of soy sauce, salt, and animal fat. Traditional or alternative ethnic foods should be used as substitutes.

Cancer

Koh, Sung, and Zhang (1996) noted that cancer ranks as a leading public health problem for Asian American and Pacific Islander populations. In the California Cancer Registry, cancer incidence and mortality rates were calculated for the six largest AAPI populations: Asian Indian, Chinese, Filipino, Japanese, Korean, and selected Southeast Asians. These women's cancer rates were similar to those for White women, with breast cancer at 28.5%, colorectal cancer at 11.9%, and lung cancer at 8.9%. However, cervical cancer (5.7%) was a problem special to AAPI women. Among AAPI males, prostate (18%), lung (17.5%), and colorectal (14.1%) cancer rates were similar to those of California White men. However, stomach and liver cancers were incidences special to AAPI men. Among AAPI men and women, lung, breast, and colorectal cancers combined were the leading causes of cancer death.

Special cancers such as liver cancer (hepatocellular carcinomas) in AAPI populations have elevated incidences for virtually all AAPI populations, primarily due to chronic hepatitis B infection in foreign-born immigrants from endemic areas. Nasopharyngeal cancer has its highest incidence rate in southern China and remains a problem for Chinese Americans. Thyroid cancer, otherwise relatively uncommon, has its highest incidence rate in Hawaii (Koh et al., 1996). Oral cavity and pharynx cancers constitute special problems for Filipino Americans.

Risk Factors.   Cancer risk factors include family history, the use of tobacco and betel nuts, and numerous nutritional factors (e.g., increased intake of meats, eggs, fat, and refined sugars).

Screening.   Screening procedures for breast cancer include mammographies and personal breast exams; for colorectal cancer, fecal occult blood tests and sigmoidoscopy; for cervical cancer, Papanicolaou (PAP) tests; for prostate cancer, rectal examinations and serum tumor markers; and for lung cancer, chest X-rays and sputum cytology.

Educating AAPI clients and families about the warning signs of cancer should be conducted in a culturally and linguistically competent manner. Nurses need to obtain patients' knowledge of cancer and understand their cultural explanations for the disease, as well as their beliefs regarding treatment. Nurses then should integrate Western beliefs of causation with beliefs held by AAPIs.

Cancer Challenges.   Koh et al. (1996) further reported that cancer issues for AAPIs present numerous ongoing challenges largely because of the extreme heterogeneity of the population. One factor to consider is the language barrier. A majority of AAPIs are immigrants; only a minority is American born, speaking English as a first language. Also, some AAPIs are children adopted from overseas. Other issues presented in cancer prevention include a lack of culturally trained healthcare providers, cost of care, and immigration status, which can restrict eligibility to public entitlement programs. Conceptual barriers—including Western and Asian knowledge of, and beliefs and attitudes about, cancer causation and early detection—also should be considered.

Hepatitis B Infection

Tong (1996) reported that studies show the prevalence of hepatitis B virus (HBV) carriers in Asian Americans range from 5% to 15%. Prevalence studies on hepatitis B antibodies indicate that 65% of Asian Americans have circulating HBV antibodies. Therefore, if one estimates the total number of

Asian Americans who are infected or who have been exposed to hepatitis B, the prevalence rate rises to 80% among Chinese and Southeast Asians and 60% among Koreans. Studies on the prevalence of hepatitis B surface antigens (HBsAg) in pregnant Asian American women indicate a carrier rate between 2% and 19%; it is 1.9% in Asians born in the United States. Those who are HBsAg positive during pregnancy infect their infant at birth; an infection at this time results in infants who become chronic carriers of the disease.

There are two medications available for immunoprophylaxis against hepatitis B. The first is hepatitis B immunoglobulin (HBIG), which contains high-titer anti-HBs and affords passive immunization. The other is the hepatitis B vaccine. Once individuals are immunized with the hepatitis B vaccine, more than 90% will produce anti-HBs, the protective antibody.

Risk Factors. Risk factors for HBV infection include the use of infecting illicit drugs, heterosexual contact with HBV-infected persons or with persons at high risk for HBV infection (e.g., drug injectors), sexual contact with multiple partners, and male homosexual activity.

Screening. Screening for HBsAg detects active (acute or chronic) hepatitis B virus (HBV) infection, and is recommended for all pregnant women at the first prenatal visit. The test is repeated in the third trimester for women who are initially HBsAg negative yet are at increased risk for HBV infection during pregnancy. Certain persons of high risk may be screened to assess eligibility for vaccinations. A variety of educational materials about hepatitis B, published in several Asian languages, is available to families.

Wang (1996) reported on the Chinatown Health Clinic in New York City, a federally funded community health center providing affordable, bilingual, and culturally competent primary care services to the Chinese community. Its effort to provide school-based hepatitis B immunization services involved community support. Local elementary school and community health center leaders, businesspersons, and public health officials participated in the on-site hepatitis screening and immunizations.

Tuberculosis

Of all the racial/ethnic groups in the United States, Asian Americans and Pacific Islanders have the highest case rates for tuberculosis (TB) per population of 100,000 (Choi, 1996). In 1993, TB case rates were 44.5 for

AAPIs compared with 3.6 for Whites, a rate 12.4 times higher. TB rates increased among AAPI, Blacks, and Hispanic populations but decreased among Whites between 1985 and 1992. AAPIs showed further increases between 1992 and 1993. Cases frequently occur among the foreign born. Choi (1996) suggested that shame, denial, and anger are issues that present additional barriers to treatment as well as language and communication issues, access to care, and myths surrounding TB.

Screening. Screening procedures for TB infection include (a) tuberculin skin testing, recommended for asymptomatic high-risk persons, and (b) Bacille Calmette-Guerin (BCG) vaccination, considered only for selected high-risk individuals such as persons infected with HIV; those having close contacts with known or suspected TB, or persons with medical risk factors associated with TB; and immigrants from countries with high TB prevalence (e.g., Africa, Asia, and Latin America) that are medically underserved and have low-income populations. Teaching clients and families about the transmission of TB and the disease process is very important.

Human Immunodeficiency Virus

Hou and Basen-Engquist (1997) studied sexual behaviors between White and AAPI adolescents to determine the risk of human immunodeficiency virus (HIV) transmission. Based on a survey of 5,385 White and 408 AAPI high school students, White students were 2.3 times more likely than AAPIs to communicate about HIV/AIDS, 2.7 times more likely to be sexually experienced, and 2.5 times more likely to use alcohol or other drugs before engaging in sexual behaviors. The authors noted that although AAPIs have a lower rate of HIV/AIDS, once they become sexually experienced, their at-risk behaviors equal those of Whites and they have an even greater number of partners when sexually active. Attention to increasing risks of AAPI adolescents indicates a further need to provide culturally appropriate HIV/AIDS prevention programs.

Loue, Lloyd, and Phoombour (1996) described one of the few reported efforts to organize AAPI groups to address HIV transmission. Factors which led to the AAPI Community AIDS Project were emphasis on community ownership, reliance on a group consensus, use of "gatekeepers" to access communities, simultaneous multilevel programming, and a view of the community as a "coordinating entity." Loue, Lloyd, and Loh (1996) further described a prevention program for AAPI healthcare workers. Specifically, the components of the training program involve (a) a symposium for the healthcare workers, (b) a culturally appropriate HIV related video for healthcare workers and their patients, (c) ongoing training, and (d) liaison and consultative services.

Risk factors for HIV are assessed by obtaining a careful sexual history and inquiring about injection drug use. Periodic screening for HIV is recommended for all persons at increased risk of infection. Clients may conceal high-risk behavior, and others (especially women in high-risk areas) may be unknowingly at risk because of an infected sex partner.

Screening. Initial screening tests to detect antibodies for HIV are enzyme immunoassay (EIA), Western blot (WB), and viral culture. Informed consent is necessary prior to HIV testing. All communications must be culturally relevant.

Mental Health

Kuramoto (1996) identified studies verifying that AAPIs have mental health problems and, in some instances, very severe mental health problems. Westermeyer, Vang, and Nieder (1984) studied Laotian Hmong refugees in Minnesota and found high rates of psychiatric disorders. Other studies found that Chinese, Japanese, Filipino, and Korean participants had higher average scores than Whites on the Center for Epidemiological Studies-Depression Scales (Kuo, 1984).

The impact of managed care on the mental health services and the types performed are of concern. Service and certification standards often discriminate and fiscally penalize AAPI providers by not acknowledging the cultural and linguistic diversity in the AAPI communities (Shinn, 1996). AAPI services are seen as "add ons" and are not integrated into the total service system. There are recommendations to broaden provisions and services for severe acculturation adjustment conditions that often exist in refugee and new immigrant populations. Shinn (1996) further noted that with the transition of mental health to managed care, "values of competition, cost containment, and financial risk adopted are in conflict with small, grass roots community-based AAPI services that stress service access, collaboration and development of indigenous professionals" (p. 208).

Diego, Yamamoto, Nguyen, and Hifumi (1994) noted that, with the influx of Asian Pacific Islanders over the years, there are increased rates of suicide among elderly Chinese and Japanese. The higher rates of suicide are due to acculturation of their children and subsequent cultural conflicts. (There *are* differences in attitudes toward suicide.) The traditional Japanese view suicide as acceptable because of their emphasis on feeling useful. For example, elderly Asians who are isolated, suffering from chronic health problems, or disabled may feel worthless or believe themselves to be a burden, and thus consider suicide. Chinese, Koreans, Filipinos, and Vietnamese are less tolerant of suicide. From 1984 to 1989, Diego et al. (1994) analyzed death certificates and coroners' files across five Asian groups; all of the deceased were over the age of 60 and living in Los Angeles County at the time of death. The researchers found that of a total of 48, the highest number of suicide victims among Asians were Japanese males, followed by Chinese and Japanese females. They concluded that culture does play a role in suicide.

Risk Factors.   Risk factors include the history of migration for certain groups such as Southeast Asians, where they have experienced the trauma of war and violence. Other risk factors identified are cultural conflicts resulting from acculturation issues between the older and younger generations. Risk factors for suicide include the presence of psychiatric illness, social adjustment problems, and serious medical illness; living alone; recent bereavement; personal or family history of suicide attempts and completed suicides; divorce and separation; and unemployment.

Screening.   Screening includes awareness of the shame and stigmas associated with mental illness. Culturally competent providers should understand that evidence of depression among AAPI groups would include expressions of somatic complaints, rather than affective symptoms, thought to be more culturally acceptable because of the shame and stigma attached to having emotional problems. Depressive symptoms can be seen particularly among adolescents and young adults; persons with a family or personal history of depression; and those with chronic illness or who have experienced recent loss, sleep disorders, chronic pain, or multiple unexplained somatic complaints (Louie, 1996).

In one early study, Yee and Lee (1977) described the development of a high school primary prevention program that provided Filipino youth with a positive view of their cultural identity. The students learned their values and behaviors differed from those of White students. They were taught to examine the strengths and resources of the Western culture to provide effective coping ability and hence positive mental health.

Tobacco Use

Tobacco use is the single most preventable cause of death and disease in this country. Reduction of cigarette smoking among Southeast Asians is a national health promotion objective for the year 2000 (DHHS, 1990). Shelton (1996) reported that cigarette smoking prevalence estimates range from 17% to 43% among AAPI men and less than 10% among AAPI women. A study released in 1993 indicated that AAPIs were the most intensely targeted ethnic groups for advertisement and promotion of tobacco use (Chen, 1994). Another study showed that tobacco billboard advertisements were highest in AAPI neighborhoods (Wildey, Young, Elder, de-Moor, Wolf, Fiske, & Sharp, 1992).

Smoking tobacco rates in Asian men are among the highest in the world. A review by Chen and Hawks (1995) showed AAPI male smoking rates were more than 50% among Southeast Asian men in the United States, compared with 25% among U.S. White males. AAPI smoking cessation initiatives have included community health center-based programs and layman-led cessation efforts conducted in several native Asian languages.

Tobacco use is a long standing and complex problem requiring multi-faceted solutions. Shelton (1996) reported six components of prevention: treatment/cessation, protection/smoke-free indoor air, counteradvertising, economic incentives, and product regulations.

Comprehensive School Health Education Programs.   Comprehensive school health education programs can reduce tobacco use among young people. Centers for Disease Control (CDC) guidelines, titled "Guidelines for school health programs to prevent tobacco use and addiction," contain key elements designed to help students develop skills in communication, problem solving, decision making, and social assertiveness; cope with anxiety; and improve their self-image (CDC, 1994). Other educational programs include enforcing school policy on tobacco use; educating youth about the physical and social consequences of tobacco use; providing a visible and reinforcing nonsmoking message to young people; providing for adequate teacher training, involving parents or guardians in support of school-based programs; supporting cessation efforts between students and school staff; and assessing the tobacco use prevention program at regular intervals.

Treatment/Cessation.   Developing and supporting interventions such as policies and enforcement initiatives may reduce youth access to tobacco products and subsequent addictions. Culturally appropriate treatment of nicotine addiction is one of the key issues addressed by tobacco prevention and control efforts in the AAPI community.

There has been an increase in the number and type of policies restricting smoking in public places, work sites, child-care facilities, schools, and hospitals.

In 1993, the tobacco companies spent $6.2 billion, or about $17 million per day, to advertise and promote their products. Increasing dollars appear to target young people, women, and minorities. Over the last thirty years, tobacco companies have significantly increased their promotional expenditures while decreasing advertising expenditures with such items as T-shirts, caps, jackets, lighters, mugs, and camping and adventure gear. Tobacco companies also have sponsored cultural, sporting, and recreational events that attract young people.

There is growth of AAPI tobacco control movements in California and Massachusetts. Lew (1996) reported that the California Asian Pacific Islander Tobacco Education Network (APITEN) and Hawaii Interagency Council on Smoking and Health led a successful campaign to defeat a tobacco industry bill that would have preempted local ordinances in Hawaii. Various Asian health services such as the Asian and Pacific Islander American Health Forum, Association of Asian Pacific Community Health Organization, National Asian Pacific American Families Against Substance Abuse, and Asian American Pacific Islander Health Promotion, together launched the first national AAPI tobacco control network, called APPEAL (Asian Pacific Partners for Empowerment and Leadership). The mission of APPEAL is to prevent tobacco use and improve health status in the AAPI community through network development, capacity building, education, advocacy, and leadership. The goal is to build and strengthen partnerships with other ethnic minority communities.

CONCLUSION

A majority of studies written about Asian American Pacific Islanders stress the need to address health promotion and disease prevention strategies in the sociocultural context of AAPIs. Nurses should be knowledgeable of the diversity among AAPI subgroups, and of language barriers, care affordability, beliefs and attitudes about health and illness, value on the integration of the mind and body, and traditional folk practices. An individual is influenced by a number of diverse cultural factors and the interaction of cultural beliefs can create barriers to compliance with recommended prevention, early detection, and screening activities (Palos, 1994). Health promotion programs must be culturally and linguistically appropriate, and healthcare providers must be knowledgeable of the cultural backgrounds. Chen (1993) noted that these interventions need to be approved by the ethnic community leaders.

Lin-Fu (1993) discussed lack of data on health problems, a healthcare issue of special concern to AAPIs. This paucity of information resulted in only identifying eight objectives targeting AAPIs of the total 336 objections in Healthy People 2000. Healthcare providers, researchers, and health policymakers must take steps toward meeting the special needs of this population and assuring culturally competent services.

REFERENCES

Casper, M., Wing S., Strogatz, D., Davis, C. E., & Tyroler, H. A. (1992). Antihypertensive treatment and US tends in stroke mortality, 1962–1980. *American Journal of Public Health, 821,* 1600–1606.

Centers for Disease Control. (1994). Prevention guidelines for school health programs to prevent tobacco use and addiction. *Morbidity and Mortality Weekly Report, 43* (No.RR-2)

Chen, M. S. (1993). A 1993 status report of the health status of APIA: Comparison with Healthy People 2000 Objectives. *Asian American and Pacific Islander Journal of Health, 1*(1), 37–55.

Chen, M. S. (1994). Failing grades given for API anti-smoking efforts. *Asian American Pacific Islander Journal of Health, 2*(1), 67–77.

Chen, M. S., & Hawks, B. L. (1995). A debunking of the myth of the healthy Asian American and Pacific Islander. *American Journal of Health Promotion, 8*(4), 261–268.

Chen, Y. L. (1996). Conformity with nature: A theory of Chinese American elders health promotion and illness prevention processes. *Advances in Nursing Science, 19*(2), 17–26.

Choi, P. (1996). Tuberculosis concerns for Asian Americans and Pacific Islanders. *Asian American and Pacific Islander Journal of Health, 4*(1/3), 127.

Diego, A. T., Yamamoto, J., Nguyen, I. H., & Hifumi, S. S. (1994). Suicide in the elderly: Profiles of Asians and whites. *Asian American and Pacific Islander Journal of Health, 2*(1), 50–57.

Enas, E. A. (1996). Cardiovascular diseases in Asian Americans and Pacific Islanders. *Asian American and Pacific Islander Journal of Health, 4*(1/3), 119–120.

Frye, B. L. (1995). Use of cultural themes in promoting health among Southeast Asians refugees. *American Journal of Health Promotion, 9*(4), 269–280.

Hou, S. I., & Basen-Engquist, K. (1997). Human immunodeficiency virus risk behaviors among white and Asian/Pacific Islander high school students in the US:
Does culture make a difference? *Journal of Adolescent Health, 20*(1), 68–74.

Koh, H., Sung, T., & Zhang, Y. Q. (1996). Cancer in Asian American and Pacific
Islander populations. *Asian American and Pacific Islander Journal of
Health, 4*(1/3), 121–124.

Kuo, W. H. (1984). Prevalence of depression among Asian Americans. *Journal of
Nervous and Mental Diseases, 172,* 449–457.

Kuramoto, F. (1996). Mental health and substance abuse: Crucial health issues
for Asian and Pacific Islander Populations. *Asian American and Pacific Islander Journal of Health, 4*(1/3), 128–130.

Lew, R. (1996). Striving toward a tobacco-free Asian American/Pacific Islander
community. *Asian American and Pacific Islander Journal of Health,
4*(1/3), 191–194.

Lin-Fu, J. S. (1993). Asian and Pacific Islander Americans. An overview of demographic characteristics and health care issues. *Asian American and Pacific
Islanders Journal of Health, 1*(1), 20–35.

Loue, S., Lloyd, L. S., & Loh, L. (1996). HIV prevention in the US Asian Pacific Islander communities: An innovative approach. *Journal of Health Care for the
Poor and Underserved.* 7(4), 364–376.

Loue, S., Lloyd, L. S., & Phoombour, E. (1996). Organizing Asian Pacific Islanders in an urban community to reduce HIV risk: A case study. *AIDS Education and Prevention, 8*(5), 381–393.

Louie, K. B. (1996). Cultural issues in psychiatric mental health nursing. In S.
Lego (Ed.), *American handbook of psychiatric nursing.* Philadelphia: Lippincott.

McGinnis, J. M., & Foege, W. H. (1993). Actual causes of death in the US. *Journal
of the American Medical Association, 270,* 2207–2212.

Palos, G. (1994). Cultural heritage: Cancer screening and early detection. *Seminars in Oncology Nursing, 10*(2), 104–113.

Pender, N. J. (1996). *Health promotion in nursing practice* (3rd ed.). Norwalk,
CT: Appleton-Century-Croft.

Shelton, D. (1996). Tobacco control issues for Asian and Pacific Islander
Americans. *Asian American and Pacific Islander Journal of Health,
4*(1/3), 185–190.

Shinn, A. (1996). Mental health concerns for Asian Americans and Pacific
Islanders. *Asian American and Pacific Islander Journal of Health,
4*(1/3), 207–208.

Tong, M. J. (1996). The impact of hepatitis B infection in Asian Americans. *Asian
American and Pacific Islander Journal of Health, 4*(1/3), 125–126.

Wang, G. (1996). Immunization concerns for Asian Americans and Pacific
Islanders. *Asian American and Pacific Islander Journal of Health,
4*(1/3), 183–184.

Westermeyer, J., Vang, T. F., & Nieder, J. (1984). Symptom change over time among Hmong refugees: Psychiatric patients versus nonpatients. *Psychotherapy, 17,* 168–177.

Wildey, M. B., Young, R. L., Elder J. P., DeMoor, C., Wolf, K. R., Fiske, K. E., & Sharp, E. (1992). Cigarette point-of-sale advertising in ethnic neighborhoods in San Diego, California. *Health Values, 16*(1), 23–28.

Yee, T. T., & Lee, R. H. (1977). Based on cultural strengths, a school primary prevention program for Asian American youth. *Community Mental Health Journal, 13*(3), 239–248.

CHAPTER TWO

The Golden Health Promotion Program for the Golden Dreamers

A. Gigi V. Moneda, MSN, ARNP

Sandra E. Gibson, EdD, ARNP

*T*he highly diverse Asian population is one of the fastest growing minorities in the United States. Data from the 1990 census documents indicate a dramatic growth in the numbers of minority Americans from 1980 to 1990 (Bryant, 1991). In addition, the percentage of minority groups 65 years and older is expected to increase approximately 20% by the year 2050 (Browne & Broderick, 1994).

The Filipino population has been moving into the United States since 1903 seeking economic and educational advantages (Melendy, 1995). Most emigrants among this industrious, family-oriented group arrived in the United States in the 1970s and 1980s. By 1990, over a million Filipinos were documented residents of the United States.

These new arrivals came predominantly as family units intending to make their homes in the urban areas of California and Hawaii. States with more than 30,000 Filipinos in 1990 include Florida, Illinois, New York, New Jersey, Texas, and Washington (Melendy, 1995).

The focus of this chapter is on the largest and most recent wave of immigrating Filipino parents who joined their children in South Florida in the 1970s and 1980s. Most of these immigrants established residence with their children who had acquired economic stability and housing. And some lived temporarily with their family in Florida while maintaining citizenship and property in the Philippines.

Many of these elderly Filipinos experienced shock and loneliness. They found themselves isolated from people familiar with the customs of their country. While their children worked, they often were left home alone. Many were given many household and babysitting tasks that were emotionally unfulfilling and often unfamiliar. Members of this elderly group often had chronic health problems that needed attention, and many felt displaced and confused. They were constantly asking their children questions about how to obtain health insurance, wanting to relieve the burden they felt they imposed on their children.

A study of this group by DiPasquale-Davis and Hopkins (1996) revealed that a majority did not have residency to qualify for Medicaid and/or Medicare. The researchers also found that should the elderly Filipinos become sick or need maintenance care for a variety of chronic conditions (i.e., hypertension, diabetes mellitus, and arthritis), health costs were usually absorbed by their children. Clearly this group of elderly needed assistance with healthcare questions and needs, along with their children. A strong point for the group was that they believed in maintaining health through exercise and diet, but they needed help remaining healthy and accessing the American health system.

WALKING DOWN A NEW ROAD: THE HEALTH PROMOTION PROGRAM

Elderly Filipinos were at a crossroad. They needed answers and were ready to start, but *how?* How would they get started? What would they focus on? Would their children help them?

They joined family and friends around living room tables covered with food. And surrounded by music, singing, dancing, merriment, and excitement, these Golden Dreamers began a project: To adapt the Health Promotion Program as part of their social support and cultural unity. Specifically, the goals were:

- To address the health maintenance needs of elderly Filipinos.
- To provide a forum for the expression of Filipino cultural diversity.

The goals and objectives have evolved since the program's creation, and today it is organized, well attended, and interactive with the community. It is important to note that the structure and development of this program started as, and continues to be, an interactive family process. This process is primarily responsible for the longevity of the program and its ability to adjust to the needs of elderly Filipinos. Objectives they thought could enhance their current health practices were identified by the elderly and their children in concert, and they follow:

- Identifying the healthcare needs of the elderly through question-naires and direct interviews.
- Maintaining a group to educate the elderly Filipinos about their acute and chronic illnesses.
- Discussing safety issues of the normal age related physical and emo-tional changes.
- Providing monthly physical and psychological screenings and com-munity referrals.
- Creating a multicultural center for Filipinos and students of other cultures to enhance their knowledge of diversity.
- Promoting multicultural learning and research.
- Obtaining at least one local grant to cover building utilization and program costs for the next five years.

Although the task was overwhelming, the timing was right. Elderly Fil-ipinos and their children, especially those who were health profession-als, were ready to strike a blow for health promotion.

The project was motivated by the loneliness that many of the elderly felt for the "old country." They loved getting together with their friends to talk, sing, eat, and dance. The socialization seemed to fill a deep need for to-getherness. As time moved on, they realized they needed a regular group of their own.

One of the elders, with the assistance of a friend, initiated the idea of having the elderly together to ease their loneliness. As founders, they talked about what was wanted by and needed for their friends, and organized a so-cial program called the Golden Dreamers Association of Miami, Florida. The association's purpose was to gather elderly Filipinos to share experi-ences regarding adjustments to the United States and provide opportunities to reminisce about the old country. Their goal in Tagalog is *Magsama-Sama, Magsaya Sa Hirap at Ginhawa,* in the founder's words, "Sharing things, having good time, happiness, and helping one another."

THE GOLDEN DREAMERS

On December 4, 1992, seven people were finally installed as Golden Dreamers. The founder appointed all officers, including a male president. The appointment of a man to the office of president was very much in line with the cultural bias that men always maintain the seat of honor. Many of the female members verbalized that they felt "a man could do a better job," as was the custom in the old country. In 1993 the founder's daughter, a health professional, started to attend the social events and observed that many of the elderly Golden Dreamers were complaining about their physical ailments and the lack of resources to access the medical system. She immediately saw the potential for health promotion, and because of her familial connection with the group, she was trusted and treated like family.

The group met every first Sunday of the month. Members would bring home-cooked food, and there would be dancing and singing, at these meetings. Charter members were strong supporters of the project and applauded participants' attendance. Consequently, response from the Filipino elderly was positive and membership rose from 7 to 65 members within the first two years.

At the beginning, one of the biggest problems was finding a place to conduct the meetings. Meetings often took place in backyards and were sometimes truncated when the hosts found they were losing their privacy. After many phone calls and prayers, a site was found: a church social hall.

Soon the group began meeting every second Sunday of the month. Health promotion sessions were held on a different day. Donations were collected and matched by a facilitator to pay for the $45-per day meeting place. This was a financial hardship since group members did not have ample financial resources.

The Golden Dreamers unanimously decided to integrate the health promotion programs with the regular meetings, which were now every first Sunday of the month.

As the program progressed, elderly Filipinos identified their need for a forum not only to socialize but also to get answers for their personal, medical, and financial dilemmas. They started a "sunshine fund," the purpose of which was to provide financial donations to those affected by illness or death. A treasurer kept record of the funds and of those who were ill.

One of the program's goals was to bring health promotion information and resources to the elderly. Access to these resources are important to ongoing medical care since many of the Golden Dreamers' financial issues were surrounding medical care costs. Thus formulating a resource for medical information, financial sources, and referrals became an essential need.

Health promotion programs consisted of educational topics ranging from the aging process, diet, and exercise, to safety and community referrals and tips on communicating needs to physicians. One of the first classes focused on exercise. Discussing and demonstrating exercise was an opportunity to translate how increased activity affected the heart, lungs, cholesterol, and weight. The program also included blood pressure screening and medication counseling. The exercise classes offered were basically calisthenics and dancing. These appealed to the Golden Dreamers because they provided an opportunity for them to get away from their home settings—away from household chores—a chance to be with friends and have fun. Many of the elderly verbalized feelings of being cared for and a sense of happiness when surrounded by their peers, and this became an effective advertisement for the program, bringing in Filipino members and volunteers.

HEALTH PROBLEMS

The morbidity and mortality of the group has been fairly low until this year (1997). Table 2.1 shows that there were three deaths over a four-year period. One of the elderly participants believed that one death from emphysema was due to poor health habits of the individual. Several of the Golden Dreamers confirmed that he "just could not stop smoking."

The morbidity data collected by the treasurer revealed that illnesses among the Golden Dreamers involved several dimensions of foundation behaviors that affect wellness (Dines, 1993). Table 2.2 contains diagnoses that suggest the Golden Dreamers may profit greatly from lifestyle changes that may conflict with many of their cultural practices.

DiPasquale-Davis and Hopkins (1996) found in their study of healthcare behaviors that many elderly Filipinos between ages 55 and 64 ate foods high in fat, exercised regularly, drank small amounts of alcohol, and used tobacco. It's interesting to note that this population stated that food was the most important contributor to good health. However, none of the elderly respondents believed their health status was excellent or good.

Table 2.1   Mortality Diagnoses for the Golden Dreamers (1994-1997)

Diagnosis	1994	1995	1996	1997
Cancer		X		
Motor vehicle accident		X		
Emphysema				X

Table 2.2   Morbidity Diagnoses for the Golden Dreamers (1994–1997)

Diagnosis	1994	1995	1996	1997
Angina	X			X
Cerebrovascular accident	X			
Falls		X (1)	X (2)	
Emphysema			X	
Abdominal surgery			X	
Peripheral vascular disease			X	
Myocardial infarction				X
Renal failure				X

HEALTHCARE ATTITUDES OF THE GOLDEN DREAMERS

Two colleagues from the school of nursing assisted in identifying health behaviors and practices of the Golden Dreamers (DiPasquale-Davis & Hopkins, 1996). These researchers were able to access the group through its monthly meetings. The findings of DiPasquale-Davis and Hopkins (1996) gave impetus to changes in the program. Since their study revealed that food and attitudes regarding personal health were problematic, they started to focus on programs that addressed these needs. A majority of the Golden Dreamers were exercising daily and did not have problems with physical activity, alcohol consumption, or tobacco use during the survey period. These behaviors were identified as minimal problems because they had been addressed in previous sessions. The elderly were praised for maintaining this important health maintenance behavior and were encouraged to continue.

THE PROGRAM

The Golden Health Promotion Program came to life during the Golden Dreamers' monthly meetings. Each begins with individual blood pressure screenings, at which time the Golden Dreamers have the opportunity to seek advice or counsel from nursing students obtaining the blood pressures. They ask questions regarding medications and illnesses they have heard about (e.g., constipation and arthritis). Educational presentations

Table 2.3   Annual Health Programs for the Golden Dreamers (1994–1997)

Month	1994	1995	1996	1997
January	Research: Findings on the Golden Dreamers	B/P Screening	Weight Control	Family First Aid
February	Glucose Screening Exercise B/P Screening	B/P Medication: Compliance	B/P Screening	B/P Screening Management of High B/P
March	Diet: Low Cholesterol, Low Fat, and Limited Salt Exercise B/P	B/P Screening	B/P	B/P Fall Prevention
April	Exercise Lecture B/P Screening	Effects of Alcohol	B/P Effects of Tobacco	B/P How to Decrease Morbidity from Falls
May	Pulse Lecture B/P Screening	B/P	B/P	B/P
June	Importance of Drinking Water B/P Screening	Effects of Tobacco	B/P Aging Process	B/P Importance of the Vaccine
July	Importance of Good Footwear during Exercise B/P Screening			B/P Management of Constipation
August	Diet Lecture B/P Screening	B/P	B/P	B/P Management of Arthritic Pain
September	Exercise B/P Screening	B/P	B/P Fall Prevention	B/P Buckle Up
October	What Is a Heart Attack B/P Screening	B/P	B/P Medication	B/P Normal Aging Process
November	B/P Screening	B/P	B/P	B/P
December	B/P	B/P	B/P Stress Reduction	B/P Stress Reduction

Note: B/P = blood pressure.

are given predominately through discussion and lectures accompanied by visual aids. A Filipino dietitian schedules individual consultations and class sessions for the entire group.

Dance classes continue to be a big hit. The elderly love the music and enjoy discussing the effects of exercise on their heart, lungs, cholesterol level, and weight. Such interests on the part of the Golden Dreamers instigated the previously mentioned blood pressure screenings, as well as counseling sessions, physical examinations, and referrals. Additionally, the elderly Filipinos were instructed on when to call for medical assistance for themselves. They also discussed what to convey to their children when they need medical help, and the children were included in sessions on the aging process and how sight and hearing affects communication.

A wide variety of topics are discussed that help the Dreamers to achieve healthy living habits (Table 2.3). Diet, exercise, medications, and safety are the primary issues addressed. Furthermore, the elderly are assisted in identifying measures and strategies to prevent illness. It is important to note that program planning is a participative activity; the Golden Dreamers are always consulted regarding program changes and development.

KEEPING THE GOLDEN DREAM ALIVE

Most of the educational programs are given in collaboration with the local chapters of nursing organizations, university faculty, undergraduate and graduate students, and community volunteers. Volunteers are solicited primarily through the Nursing Student Organization, which is headed by a student leader. Oftentimes, the family, friends, and colleagues assist or present programs. The volunteer component is working very well; recruitment is not problematic. The volunteers seem to love coming back. They voice that the experience is very insightful and effects a positive change on the way they practice nursing by enhancing their level of understanding of and sensitivity to other cultural groups.

Golden Dreamers show their support by contributing dues for the social hall and maintaining a very high attendance. And their families help by volunteering their time to make copies of handouts, carry equipment to and from the church, and even attend meetings.

Several donations have been contributed by community supporters. A private laboratory sponsored cholesterol screening tests for the entire group. A local physician agreed to manage those Dreamers with a history of hypertension and accepted referrals from the cholesterol screening. Moreover, this same physician accepted a limited number into a national hypertension study. Through this study, they were able to obtain free medical care including medication. And the same physician continues to contribute his time and expertise as the unofficial medical director of the Golden Health Promotion Program.

The Philippine Nurses Association of Florida assists with health screenings and pledges to adapt the Golden Health Promotion Program as one of its local community projects. Other invaluable benefactors include allied health professionals (e.g., dietitians), undergraduate and graduate nursing students, and nursing faculty from local universities.

Presently, the Golden Dreamer Health Promotion Program is moving into its third year of operation and showing no signs of slowing down. The Golden Dreamers have become a presence in the Filipino community, and it is anticipated that funding will soon be a worry of the past.

FUTURE GOLDEN DREAMS

Future horizons for the Golden Dreamers look clear and bright. The timing is right to explore funding for long-term support of the Golden Dreamers' social and educational programs. It is time to move beyond the small donations of the immediate community and search for funding that will not only include the elderly Filipinos but also the entire family system. Expanding services to Golden Dreamers' children and their offspring—the group's most recent vision—calls for a holistic health promotion program to be experienced in the House of the Golden Dreamers. The House would be open for all of the Filipino community and individuals who want to learn about Filipino culture. The House of the Golden Dreamers will be a place for education, mutual support, cultural enrichment, safety, and expressions of cultural memories and pride.

A very special part of the project should evolve to provide special support for new arrivals and those seeking remembrances of the Philippines. Perhaps the center will become one of the premier multicultural centers in Miami. Financial support may be obtained from federal and corporate grants, private benefactors as well. Also, the ongoing support of the academic community, along with the community at large, would promote the mission of diversity education and give credibility to the program as an important aspect of community pride and growth.

REFERENCES

Babcock, D. E., & Miller M. A. (Eds.). (1994). *Client education: Theory & practice.* St. Louis, MO: Mosby.

Browne, C., & Broderick, A. (1994). Asian and Pacific Island elders: Issues for social work practice and education. *Social Work, 39*(3), 252–259.

Bryant, B. E. (1991, March). *The 1990 census and implications of change.* Paper presented at a meeting "Population Association of America," Washington, DC.

DiPasquale-Davis, J., & Hopkins, S. (1996). Health behaviors of an elderly Filipino group. *Public Health Nursing, 14*(2), 118–122.

Melendy, H. B. (1995). Filipino Americans. In J. Galens, A. Sheets, & R. Young (Eds.), *Gale encyclopedia of multicultural America* (pp. 499–515). Detroit, MI: Gale Research.

CHAPTER THREE

Xi Young Hong: Health Practice in Chinese Older Women

Lin Zhan, PhD, RN

*T*he rapidly increasing older population has brought new challenges and demands to the healthcare system in the United States. Of the estimated 31 million elderly people, 80% have at least one chronic condition (National Center for Health Statistics, 1990), making this group the heaviest user of health services. According to notable sources, the elder population now consumes 30% of national health funds and 50% of the federal health budget (Harris, 1990; U.S. Special Committee on Aging, 1991). Given this total demand on the healthcare system, it is imperative to determine measures for immediate implementation that can relieve both the national fiscal burden and encourage personal health. The importance of health promotion and disease prevention cannot be overestimated in this regard. Nonetheless, minority research has been and continues to be focused on "deficits" or "problems," with only a paucity of research on health promoting behaviors, especially in regard to the Chinese elderly woman.

THE STUDY

Aging is a universal phenomenon. From a biological perspective, aging is conceptualized as a process of changing functional capacities of vital organism systems. Socially, aging is described in relation to how people take, make, and play their roles in a given society and how a given society or environment impacts on individuals as they advance in age. Psychologically, aging relates to changes in one's behavioral patterns over time.

From traditional Chinese perspectives, old age itself has been considered as an "accumulation of wisdom" and the "fulfillment of happiness." *Xi Young Hong,* a Chinese common saying, refers to the time of sunset (an analogy to aging), which brings with it a bright red color to symbolize happiness. Here, health is the foremost indicator of happiness in one's later life. To bring *Xi Young Hong,* many Chinese elderly pay attention to their body and mind. But does this take place with Chinese elderly in the United States? What do they do to promote their health in a culture that is so different from their own? With these questions in mind, I conducted a qualitative study that investigated health practice among Chinese elderly women, along with facilitators and barriers in relation to health promotion in Chinese elderly women.

Method

Sample. A convenient and purposive sample consisted of 10 Chinese elderly women who reside in an urban area in the northeastern part of the United States. Sample criteria for inclusion included individuals who were age 60 or older, and had no cognitive impairment. Participants were recruited from a local Chinese community. I introduced the purpose of the study to participants at the time of recruitment, obtaining informed consent prior to each interview. I contextualized the entire study within the purview of two major research questions: What measures were used by Chinese older women to promote their health, and what were facilitators and barriers regarding health promotion among Chinese older women?

Participants' ages ranged from 72 to 89 years; the average sample age was 74. Five of the 10 were widowed, 1 was divorced, and 4 were married. Half of the total sample had education at the high school level. Eight of the women had an annual income of less than $7,999; one reported between $10,000 and $12,000, and another had an income of roughly $25,000. With respect to living arrangements, 6 of the participants lived alone; 4 lived with their spouse. Most ($n = 8$) lived in government subsidized housing which enabled them to pay for rent at less than the prevailing market price, a benefit based on the Section 202 Direct Loan Program of the Housing Act (Hooyman & Kiyak, 1933). All study participants (Table 3.1) experienced at least one chronic disease condition: diabetes ($n = 3$), visual or hearing impairment ($n = 6$), arthritis ($n = 9$), hypertension ($n = 4$), or cancer ($n = 1$).

Table 3.1   Study Sample Characteristics

Demographic Variables	Value
Ethnic Background	
Chinese American	10
Age Range	72–89
Marital Status	
Married	4
Separated or divorced	1
Widowed	5
Education	
Some high school	3
High school	5
Some college	2
Income	
Under $7,999	8
$8,000–$19,999	1
$20,000–$39,999	1
Living Arrangement	
Alone	6
With others	4
Chronic Conditions	
Arthritis	9
Hypertension	4
Visual and hearing impairment	5
Cancer	1
Diabetes	3

Data Collection.   All data came through semi-structured interviews of approximately two and one-half hours in which I asked such questions as:

- Tell me about your health.
- What have you done in promoting your health?
- What factors help you in promoting your health?
- What has been difficult for you in promoting your health?

Interviews took place at a participant's apartment ($n = 8$), a community senior center ($n = 1$), and via telephone ($n = 1$).

Participants also completed three survey questionnaires at the end of each interview. The demographic profile included information about age, education, marital status, income, and living arrangement. The 36-item

Health Status Questionnaire (HSQ) assessed multidimensions of health status concerning general health perceptions, functional status, and personal well-being, with reliability (a .88–.92) as reported by previous and present studies (Interstudy, 1991; Ware, 1986; Zhan, 1993). The 15-item Geriatric Depression Scale (GDS) was used to screen depression status, with reliability supported by a Cronbach's alpha coefficient of .94 and a one-week test–retest reliability of .85. The construct validity of the GDS was supported by evidence that known groups of normal, depressed, and severely depressed older people had significantly higher GDS mean scores, ordered as expected (Sheikh & Yesavage, 1986). Since most Chinese elderly in this study spoke little or no English ($n = 9$), I translated survey questionnaires into Chinese. To ensure further accuracy, translated documents were verified through a professional translator.

Data Analysis. I analyzed interview content data using a constant comparison method. After each in-depth interview, data transcription was conducted with substantive coding and data reduction, thereby summarizing the substance of the interview without imposing theoretical construction on the data. In the interviews I extracted significant statements and identified the meaning of each, thereafter organizing clusters of themes and core data categories. Finally, I used descriptive and correlative statistics for analysis of the normative and demographic data.

Findings and Discussion

Chinese elderly women in this study defined health in several ways: doing things one desires to do, being able to enjoy one's life, and searching for harmony between person and environment. Sample comments were: "Without health, how can you enjoy your life?" "Health, to me, means to be able to get around." "I have arthritis. But I am able to get around, to visit my friend, to cook for my children when they come, and to go fishing with my husband. I am healthy." "I am healthy as long as I feel peace and harmony." The majority of the participants rated their health status as good or excellent, despite the chronic conditions they experienced. Their judgments concerning health may be associated with how much their life is interrupted by health problems. One participant said, "Considering my health I think I am OK. I still can do things I want to do." Positive health ratings also may be related to one's expectation of health, comparison of health to that of peers, perception of health. One noted, "I have arthritis. . . .

Compared to my friend who had Parkinson's, I think I am healthy." Older people may expect a decline in their health as they age, but when the deterioration does not take place at the rate or to the extent they expected, they assess their health more positively. The result of a statistical analysis in this study supported interview data. There were significant correlations between the mean scores of the GDS and the HSQ subscale "functional status" in this sample ($r = .39$, $p < .001$), suggesting that functional status is an indicator of mental outlook. In this regard, timely interventions such as facilitating effective coping strategies and social support may be needed as the Chinese elderly experience a decline in physical functions.

One study result, Chinese elderly women showed higher GDS mean scores ($\bar{x} = 3.11$, $p < .01$), indicated a possible depression status. Although a previous study (Yu, Liu, & Kurzeja, 1985) reported that Chinese older women had the highest suicide rate of any ethnic group in the United States, contributing factors were not and have not been fully explained. Traditional Chinese culture, of course, may play a role in this distressing phenomenon, for women especially are not encouraged to disclose their feelings to family members and friends, or to seek professional therapeutic services. To be socially sensitive, personal conflicts are not expressed and are to be avoided if they disturb the harmony between the person and environment or among persons. As a result, Chinese older women may hide their feelings, so as to maintain harmony in their family and social relations. Mental problems also may be viewed as a social disgrace since Chinese philosophy emphasizes mental strength as a typical survival mechanism. Within the context of traditional beliefs, Chinese older women may experience depression but go undiagnosed and untreated. Regular depression screening for Chinese elderly women is recommended, so that appropriate and timely social and health service interventions and informal social support from family, friends, and the church can be received. Here, it is clearly a matter of life *and* health.

Health Promoting Measures

In terms of health promotion, the Chinese women in the study identified five unique measures: exercise, regular checkups, education, involvement, and the balance of *yin* and *yang*. Facilitating factors that promoted health included medical insurance, social support, and spirituality. Barriers that impeded health promotion involved language and transportation difficulties, poverty, and cultural conflict.

Exercise. Most of the women described "using your body"—"you got to move everyday"—as a way to maintain and promote their health. One elderly woman said, "I walk 1,000 steps in my apartment every day. I do not have an exercise machine. Well, what I can do is to walk three times a day, after each meal. Chinese people say 'you live up to ninety-nine years if you walk 99 steps after every meal.' That is what I am doing." Another woman told me, "I stretch [my] arms and legs several times a day." Several of the women mentioned doing Tai Chi, a traditional Chinese exercise involving a series of slow movements that require body and mind concentration. An 85-year-old woman, who lived on the eighth floor of her apartment building, walked up and down the stairwell every day. "I do not take the elevator," she said. "I go downstairs and upstairs by foot. It is a good exercise. As long as I can climb stairs, why not to do so?"

Regular Checkup. As a way to offer baseline health data the regular physical checkup was also seen as a way to keep from getting sick. One elderly woman put it this way,

> *We have nurses and doctors coming to this building regularly. The building manager makes sure that we all know that. Whenever they come, I make sure I get the physical checkup. The only problem is that I do not speak English. If the building manager is here, he helps. If he is not there, I just guess. I know I am fine if I see doctors and nurses smiling. . . . and I try to have a physical exam every year.*

However, interviews revealed that most of the elderly women did not receive comprehensive health services such as dental and mammographic exams. In terms of the latter, several women felt that they did not understand mammography enough or its diagnostic significance; for the former, they indicated not having enough money to pay for some dental expenses. One woman, while she visited her family in Shanghai, had her denture fixed and periodontal treatment done for a total cost of $50. "There is no way for me to pay these kind of treatments here," she said, smiling.

Education. Self-education was considered as an important measure to maintain health. One woman said, "You got to know what is going on inside of your body." Another woman said, "I do not like to go on without knowing whether I have problems or not . . . Sometimes it might be too late when I had symptoms." A third woman said, "You got to educate yourself, read books and newspaper. I read Chinese newspaper every Sunday since it has an entire column on health. I did not know diabetic diet before. I read a paper which answered many of my questions. It helped." Another woman said, "If you are educated you know what kind of question you need to ask your doctor." And, a fifth woman told me, "I keep my eyes and ears open to when and where I can get a flu shot. I have not had the flu for several years." Certainly self-education here implies determination to take charge of one's health and to become an educated healthcare consumer. Nurses can reinforce this health promoting behavior by providing timely, adequate, accurate, and linguistically appropriate health information to Chinese elderly and by encouraging them to assume a greater responsibility for promoting their own health.

Involvement. Some elderly women in the study were involved in community, church, and family activities, which helped them cope with their loneliness, increased their sense of involvement and self-esteem, contributed to their wisdom, and served as a form of continuity for their productive roles. One participant noted that she kept herself busy by doing volunteer work at the community senior center after her husband passed away. Others indicated that they reached out to other Chinese elderly through church activities. "I go to church every week where I met people, made new friends, and offered help if needed," said one woman. Another told me, "I keep myself very busy, calling my friends and helping out if I can." Some women preferred to be their own self-companion, to be involved in independent activities such as reading and cooking. One 89-year-old woman said, "I keep myself very busy and feel I have a lot of things to do every day. I paint, water flowers and plants, cook, do exercise, read, lots of things."

Balanced Yin *and* Yang. Balancing *yin* and *yang* has been a traditional health belief of many Chinese. According to this belief, every phenomenon is divided into two contrary components: the yin and yang, or male/female, positive/negative, day/night, and health/illness. The qualities of yin and yang are relative, not absolute. For example, the surface of the body is yang and the interior is yin. Life and death belong to yang, whereas growth belongs to yin. Yin and yang react to each other, producing change. This changing rhythm is then balanced, the yin and yang ensuring there is no excess of either; for any overactivity of yang, there is an adjustment by the yielding passivity of yin. Yin represents a cold energy force and yang, a hot energy force (Zhan, 1992). For many Chinese, diseases can come from what one eats. Eating certain foods thus can bring about a state of balance or imbalance. Here, cold and solid foods, such as

melons and raw vegetables, are used to treat hot ailments including constipation, hypertension, and sore throat. The majority of the older women
in this study viewed "eat right" as a way to balance yin and yang and
hence promote their health. Sample comments ranged from "I just pay a
lot of attention to what I eat," to "Eat regular, simple, a lot of vegetables
. . . that is good for me." One woman even mentioned her husband. "My
husband has hypertension. He needs to eat cold food rather than hot food.
In summer, we eat yin food, watermelon and vegetables. In winter, we eat
soup a lot. When I have fever, I eat cold food."

Facilitators

The Chinese elderly women in the study identified three unique facilitators to promote health: medical insurance, social support, and spirituality. All participants expressed gratitude to the Medicare or Medicaid they
received, which covered basic healthcare costs. Eighty percent of the
Chinese elderly were recipients of Medicare, Medicaid, and Supplemental
Social Income (SSI), though 9 out of the 10 in the study did not have a
working history in the United States. They lived on either their spouse's
limited pension of social security or on SSI. Mrs. Wang, for example, is 87
years old and has multiple chronic disease conditions (hypertension, osteoporosis, diabetes, and breast cancer). Her only income, from her husband's social security, was about $500 a month, or $6,000 a year, placing
her well below the poverty level of $7,360 a year. With the help of SSI and
Medicaid, she received an extra $100 per month. She no longer had to pay
expensive premiums for private insurance to supplement her Medicare
coverage. SSI also payed her monthly premium of $46 for Medicare. All
benefits combined lifted Mrs. Wang slightly above the federal poverty
level. Mrs. Wang spoke, "Without these benefits, I am not sure whether I
am still alive . . . I am very grateful."

   According to study participants, social support varied in terms of
sources, including family (mostly daughters), friends, church acquain-
tances, community services, and neighbors (see Yu & Wu, 1985; Yu et al.,
1985, for comparable study results). Central to the traditional philosophy
of Confucianism, which promotes strong social and family bonds, Chinese elderly are revered and respected. Essentially, age equals dominance
(Chae, 1987). For years it has been the Chinese custom for extended families to live together. With more and more young couples preferring to live
on their own, however, this custom has dissipated in the United States,

leaving more older people alone. Despite the daughters' role in caring and helping, Chinese elderly still wished that their children could spend more time with and live closer to them. As one woman expressed, "I wish my daughter and son spend more time with me. What can you do here? Everyone has to work hard to survive." In order to maintain ethnic values and customs, Chinese elderly tend to seek informal social support from people of their own age and the same ethnic identity in a local church or community senior center. One woman uttered, "Some of my friends died. I have to make new friends. New friends are important since you cannot depend on your children here." One participant lived in a community where she received an array of services including emergency food when needed and community assistant programs for the elderly Chinese. She said, "I come to the senior center everyday, to have my lunch here and meantime help the center cook and prepare meals for others. Here I met new friends and I called some of them everyday. We check on each other to make sure that we are OK, that is assuring."

Chinese elderly noted spirituality as an important way to promote their mental well-being. The philosophies of Confucianism and Taoism, for example, were followed to varying degrees by some women in the study. From the ancient philosophy of Tao also comes the concept of yin and yang, the two energies that must be balanced for the body to function properly—the perpetually changing rhythm of movement is an interplay that produces growth, transformation, and death (O'Hara & Zhan, 1994). According to Confucianism, one must search for harmony between person and environment and eschew excess, which prompts disturbance to the equilibrium. Balance requires harmony in self, family, and society. Sample responses included these perceptions: "I have to search for harmony and meaning in life." "I try to maintain balance mentally and physically." "You got to balance yourself to nature." "I keep close relationship with myself and do a lot of meditation . . . keep myself peaceful and calm."

Barriers

Of the barriers that impeded the Chinese elderly women from promoting their health, language was a major concern. Because most Chinese elderly in the study had difficulty in speaking and understanding written English, it tended to keep them from discussing their health problems with physicians, nurses, and other health professionals; this further limited their access to healthcare services. In one case, Mrs. Lee said, "I found bleeding when I had a bowel movement. I worried and wanted to talk to my doctor. I do not know English. My daughter is far away and she has to make long-distance phone call which is expensive since she has little money. I do not want to bother her. But I worry about my bleeding problem. I hope it is not a serious problem."[1] Language as a barrier is further exemplified in another case. Mrs. Chan's husband has had Parkinson's for two years and his condition has been deteriorating. Mrs. Chan desperately needed home care service but did not know where or how to find service resources since she spoke no English. As she said: "It is hard for me even to ask for help. I do not speak English. We are supposed to get government subsidized housing but I do not even know how to start . . . I am so worried, could not sleep, eat, and have lost several pounds. My daughter lives in another country. She tries to help but it is hard . . . I do not know what I should do? . . . I am so frightened."[2] Ironically, Mrs. Chan lived in the same community where health and social services were ample. Due to the language barrier, Mrs. Chan had no access to service information.

Another language difficulty concerns the multiplicity of Cantonese dialects spoken by most Chinese who immigrated from the southern part of China prior to the 1960s. Most participants in the study, for instance, immigrated after the 1960s and spoke only Mandarin. When they asked for a translator from the doctor's office, a Cantonese-speaking person was likely to be arranged. One woman commented, "I find the Cantonese even more difficult to understand than English. English, I may pick up some words; for Cantonese, there is no way for me to know."

As exemplified in these cases, language difficulties raise a question for nurses and health professionals: How can we reach out to non-English speaking elderly patients? Older immigrants are different from younger immigrants; they may not easily give up their traditional values and find it difficult to master another language. Because of unfamiliarity with the non-Chinese environment, most Chinese elders in the study preferred to stay near Chinatown where they could speak their own language, eat the food of their culture, and consult with herbalists or Chinese doctors. To reach out to non-English speaking elderly, community service information must be translated into the appropriate languages. It is imperative as well for health professionals to assess local dialects so that translators can

---

[1] After the interview, I helped Mrs. Lee to make an appointment with her doctor.
[2] The researcher discussed the case with a local community health nurse who then coordinated care for Mrs. Chan's family. Mrs. Chan and her family now live in the community's elderly housing and receive home care services.

be arranged for the facilitation of effective communications. Knowledge of cultural perspectives of a community sensitizes nurses to that population's needs and increases accessibility of health services to ethnic minorities (Spector, 1996).

Transportation problems generally hindered the study's participants in seeking out health services. As several pointed out, "I have to depend on a bus. I do not drive." "Transportation is a problem. I have to depend on my children to drive me to my doctor's office. When my children are not available, I have to cancel my appointment." "I go everywhere by foot. I rarely use public transportation. . . . I do not understand English and often end up riding a wrong bus or subway. In winter, it is too cold to walk around." Although some communities offer transportation services, it is uncertain how much information about the service reaches the non-English speaking elderly. For those Chinese elderly in the study, familiarity with available transportation services in the city was limited. Add to this their adhesion to nearby ethnic enclaves—Chinatown, or their own apartment—and service availability decreases even more.

Several Chinese elderly expressed their conflict between choosing Western medicine and tradition Chinese medicine. Two women who immigrated to the United States in the 1950s retained traditional beliefs more than those who immigrated after the 1970s, when the Western culture had become more widely accepted in China. Traditional Chinese medicine includes herbal remedy, diet therapy, use of animal secretion and organs, acupuncture, massage, moxibustion (the application of a burning moxa plant to skin), and other folk methods. As one participant described it, "I was given several medications for my hypertension when I visited my doctor. I came home and took Chinese medicine because it worked before when I had a symptom. I also take ginseng, which was good for my arthritis. . . . I am not sure whether I shall take Chinese medicine while taking Western medications. Sometimes I take both." Herbal medicines have been used for centuries in China, and there are thousands of herbs sent to the United States, mostly for sale in Chinatown. Ginseng root, for example, is widely used for arthritis, back pain, fatigue, and sores. Gensing, however, has been found to cause over medication in a client already taking antihypertentives (Louie, 1985). It is thus critical for nurses to assess the Chinese client thoroughly, with special attention given to knowing whether the client takes herbs and how much the client understands about the usage of Western medicines and their adverse affects. Again, language may be a factor preventing the Chinese client from asking questions regarding prescribed medications, and thus taking both Chinese herbs and Western medicines with possible adverse effects.

Another cultural conflict concerns the power relationship between provider and patient, specifically whether it is proper to challenge an expert (i.e., their doctors or nurses). If there are misunderstandings or misgivings with a prescribed regimen, Chinese elderly may not verbalize their concerns for fear of public conflict. Instead, they may return home and not follow the regimen, which can possibly raise risk factors. For example, one study participant recalled:

> One day I had an eye surgery. After surgery, I was in a waiting room. I waited for a while. Then I decided to go home. I did not understand what they told me, neither I asked them. I walked back to my apartment. I felt so tired, and then I passed out on the street. A friend of mine passed by and took me home. Usually, it takes me 15 minutes from the hospital to my apartment. This time it took me three hours.

This case exemplified that language difficulty and a cultural conflict by not questioning health professionals resulted in an increased risk factor regarding one's safety. Therefore, it is important for nurses and health professionals to know to what extent the patient speaks English, what Chinese dialect is spoken, and whether the client feels comfortable enough to ask questions. In this regard, it is especially important never to *assume* that a Chinese client understands a specific regimen, prescription use, or other health factors.

The majority of Chinese elderly identified a further barrier in health promotion: financial difficulty. As indicated, in the study 80% of the Chinese American elderly lived in poverty. Despite benefits received under Medicare and Medicaid, gaps in health coverage continue to exist. Personal payments for certain prescription drugs, eye glasses, hearing aids, dentures, and so on were difficult if not impossible. The choice was often between obtaining necessities for living or paying for uncovered health related costs. One woman said, "Sometimes, I have to choose between food and medicine." Divorce or widowhood has also had a disproportionately negative effect on the economic well-being of elderly women. One older Chinese, for example, had to receive welfare after divorcing her husband. She said, "I was OK before the divorce. Now I have to depend on welfare to survive." We cannot forget that, according to the Census Bureau (1990), two-thirds of older women who live alone are poor, and older minority women who live alone form the poorest groups in the United States.

CONCLUSION

Study findings indicate that the meaning of health is embedded in people's lives. Understanding how Chinese elderly perceive their own health is an important step in the initial assessment of clients. Along with an accurate assessment of cultural factors must come an assessment of cultural differences when designing individual or community-based health promotion programs for older patients. Identifying support sources for each ethnic group will help community health nurses, for instance, to integrate them into care. Peer support also may well serve in maintaining elderly Chinese ethnic identity within their experience of the conflict in values that earlier or more recent immigration has brought them, especially in terms of their children's lives in the United States (in the nuclear family and espousal of individuality) in contrast to the tradition of filial piety.

Health promotion and disease prevention denote comprehensive care that provides not only health services but also a means of access to these services that includes, but is not limited to, transportation, translation, education, and myriad forms of social and spiritual supports for individuals and their families, groups, aggregates, and community populations. That older Chinese in the present study experienced language difficulties, lack of familiarity with Western medicine and practice, transportation difficulties, and poverty, speak to the need to ensure and expand current health services and supports. Social isolation and immobility, limited accessibility to health and social services, and a resulting increase in health risk factors will require that nurses understand how these conditions influence health and shape disease. Programs to improve access and usage of preventive services for ethnic elderly are critical, but must also be linguistically appropriate and culturally sensitive with service information disseminated through community outreach efforts. Health professionals cannot address health promotion as a concept without also addressing access and barriers to it. Tolerating the association between social factors and health problems can only indicate our failure to identify risk factors and intervene effectively.

In regard to health policy, nurses can advocate maintaining and expanding current financial mechanisms for health promotion. There is no doubt that Medicare and Medicaid programs have increased access to healthcare for older people. Nonetheless, support for these valuable programs is being whittled away. The 1996 laws that changed SSI benefits for non-citizens have already had a devastating impact on older legal immigrants who rely heavily on SSI and Medicaid to pay for basic food, housing, and health-care needs. Nurses must advocate to keep cutbacks in Medicare and Medicaid legislation to a minimum, as well as support efforts that modulate the effects of welfare reform on non-citizens.

Health promotion exists to keep people well. Culturally sensitive approaches that minimize language barriers, engage ethnic elderly in familiar and acceptable health promoting activities, and empower them to take control over their health are essential. Access to appropriate and acceptable healthcare, a safe and healthy physical and social environment in which to promote health, and a financial floor to support healthy lifestyles will ultimately promote quality of life for all older people.

REFERENCES

Chae, M. (1987). Older Asians. *Journal of Gerontological Nursing, 13*(11), 10–17.

Harris, D. K. (1990). *Sociology of aging.* New York: Harper & Row.

Hooyman, N. R., & Kiyak, H. A. (1993). *Social gerontology* (3rd ed.). Boston: Allyn & Bacon.

Interstudy Outcome Management System. (1991). The health status questionnaire. *The Interstudy Quality Edge, 1,* 1.

Louie, K. (1985). Providing health care to Chinese clients. *Topics in Clinical Nursing, 7*(3), 18–25.

National Center for Health Statistics. (1990). *Health United States, 1989 and prevention profile* (DHHS Publication No. PHS 90-1232). Hayttsvile, MD: Author.

O'Hara, E. M., & Zhan, L. (1994, October). Cultural and pharmacological considerations when caring for Chinese elders. *Journal of Gerontological Nursing,* 11–16.

Sheikh, J. I., & Yesavage, J. A. (1986). Geriatric depression scale: Recent evidence and development of a shorter version. *Clinical Gerontologist, 5*(1/2), 165–173.

Spector, R. (1996). *Cultural diversity in health and illness.* Stamford: Appleton & Lange.

U.S. Census Bureau. (1990). *Money income and poverty status in the United States. Current population reports* (Series P-60, No. 168). Washington, DC: U.S. Government Printing Office.

U.S. Senate Special Committee on Aging. (1991). *Aging: Aging Americans, trends and projections.* Washington, DC: Author.

Ware, J. E. (1986). The assessment of health status. In L. Aiken & D. Mechanic (Eds.), Application of filial belief and behavior within the contemporary Chinese American family. *International Journal of Sociology of the Family, 13,* 17–36.

Yu, E. S. H., Liu, W. T., & Kurzeja, P. K. (1985). Physical and mental health status indicators for Asian-American communities. *Reports of the Secretary's Task Force on black and minority health. Vol. II. Cross-cutting issues in minority health* (pp. 255-283). Rockville, MD: U.S. Department of Health and Human Services.

Yu, L. C., & Wu, S. C. (1985). Unemployment and family dynamics in meeting the needs of Chinese elderly in the United States. *Gerontologists, 25,* 474-476.

Zhan, L. (1992). *Functional health pattern assessment: Chinese perspectives.* Unpublished manuscript, Boston College School of Nursing.

Zhan, L. (1993). *Cognitive adaptation process in the hearing-impaired elders.* Doctoral dissertation, Boston College.

PART II

Healthcare and Health Related Issues

CHAPTER FOUR

Korean Women and Health

Kyung Rim Shin, EdD, RN

*T*he health of women in Korea is an important foundation for their lives, their families, and their society. Women are the "center of health." They are important in the determination of a healthy environment and a lifestyle that affects their domestic roles and the health of their children. However, because women have been socially placed in a secondary position, the concrete, integrative, and progressive emphasis on their health has been limited to an itemized discussion of their health problems.

Until now, women's health generally has been discussed in terms of generative problems. This is because women are not considered independent personalities, but are believed to be procreational vehicles. Today women's lives are changing in accordance with the surrounding social, economical, and cultural changes.

In Korea, women have more health problems, attend hospitals more frequently, and need more medical treatment than men. There are few adequate institutional medical services for women. As a result, women seek and have become dependent on uncommon medical cures.

Women are different from men in their physical frame, strength, and body structure. Pregnancy and birth, puerperal complications, contraception, abortion, menstruation, and physiological cancer or infection are a few examples of health problems experienced by women.

Lately, the patriarchal culture, which seeks to rationalize men's possession and domination of women, has begun to change. Yet sexual violence against women and prostitution are prevalent in Korean society; accordingly, sexually transmitted diseases, including acquired immunodeficiency syndrome (AIDS), have surfaced collectively as a Korean social problem.

Chronic geriatric diseases also are found more frequently among women than men. This occurrence is not only because of changes in women's lifestyles, but also because of an increasing population of aging women, who outlive men by an average of 8 years. Women, especially, show a high ratio of degenerative musculoskeletal and coronary circulatory diseases.

Korean women tend to be quite anxious and feel deeply threatened by social prejudices. Traditionally, women were compelled to take exclusive responsibility for housework and nursing. Women who participated in social work, or younger women, felt that the role they had to play in housework, nursing, and family relations was a heavy psychological burden. Today's Korean society, still influenced by sex-role obsessions, denies women's self-esteem, adhering to the conventional "good wife," "wise mother" roles, rather than trying to understand women's lives and their experiences. As a result, a large number of women have mental disorders. They internalize their psychological troubles and withdraw into a self-contradicting state.

Moreover, women's health is closely related to the development of their society and country.

> *Women's health is a unified part of the whole development of her country, and therefore it depends highly on what stage her country's development is situated in. Therefore the advance of women's health is at first hand a contribution to the economic and social development of her country, and at second hand a contribution for the health and welfare of her family. (Sterm, 1996)*

Women's health can be largely defined as a state of their holistic development. The quality of women's lives is capable of improvement: Women can maintain healthy lifestyles; participate in a productive social role; develop their abilities; and live satisfactory lives. But in order to achieve these goals, it is essential that they receive various material and institutional support from their families and society.

The development of women includes improvements in health, acquisition of social capability, and attainment of social support. The Fourth World Women's Conference, held in Beijing in 1995, announced a code of conduct composed of 22 provisions and 5 strategy targets, all concerning women and their health. At this conference, women's health was defined as a "state of physical, mental, and social well-being, not just an absence of disease or ailment. It includes emotional, social, and physical welfare, and is determined not only by biology but also by social, political, and economic life" (World Health Organization, 1988). Women's health should be an integrative state of physical, mental, social, economical, intellectual, and spiritual well-being.

This chapter examines the health of Korean women by exploring their demographic characteristics and health problems, and the medical services provided for them. It also proposes suggestions for the improvement of women's health.

DEMOGRAPHIC CHARACTERISTICS

Movement in Population

The population of Korea is expected to increase from 1995's 45,090,000 to 50,620,000 by 2010, and reach 52,740,000 in 2030. Growth of the population will decline from a yearly average of 0.9% to 0.6% between 2005 and 2010, falling to an average of 0.1% between 2020 and 2030.

Due to a declining birthrate, the number of infants and children will decrease while that of older people will increase. The population growth rate of infants and children is projected to decrease from 1995's 23.4% to 19.9% by 2010, to 16% by 2030. On the other hand, the population growth rate of elders over age 65 will increase from 1995's 5.9% to 7.1% by 2000, developing a society of people in advanced age and reaching a rapid growth rate of 19.3% in 2030 (National Statistical Office, 1996).

The life span of Koreans increased between the mid-1970s and 1995. The average life span of women is 77.4 years, and the life span of men is age 68.6. However, the life span of good health for women is age 49.9; for men, 50.7. This record shows that women suffer from illness for an average of 25 years throughout their lives and men suffer for an average of 16 years. The average span of health that excludes barriers of action stops at age 62.6.

The population consisting of people at ages capable of conception (ages 15–64) will increase from 1995's 70.7% to 71.2% by the year 2000, but will afterwards decrease to 70.2% by 2010, then to 64.7% by 2030. Maintenance of such a low birthrate will increase the average life span. The number of youngsters will decrease while the number of elders will increase, resulting in a short labor supply through the years 2000 to 2010.

Infertility. The population of women capable of conception (ages 15–64), which influences the population of newborns, is expected to increase from 1995's 12,860,000 to 13,400,000 by the year 2000, and then gradually decline to 1,083,000 by 2030. The population of people ages 20 to 34, those who are likely to conceive children, was 6,310,000 in 1995. But this number is projected to decline to 4,650,000 by 2030. This decrease will accordingly bring a decline in the population of newborns.

Increase of Single Women.   The rate of families constituting one person (a one-person family) has increased greatly since 1980, from 4.8% to 9.0% in 1990, and to 12.7% in 1995. Reasons for this increase include a higher average age at marriage and the migration of young people from the rural regions to the cities.

The rate of unmarried women ages 25 to 29 increased from 1985's 18.4% to 22.1% in 1990, but between the years 1990 and 1995, the rate suddenly increased to 29.9%. Even with improved education levels and development of economic activities, this was a very rapid increase. If the older age group also should increase at such a rapid rate, it is certain to influence the decline of the birth rate.

Increase of Divorced Women.   The divorce rate in Korea has been increasing. Research showed that the total number of divorced couples has been increasing in geometrical progression, from 11,625 in 1970 to 22,980 in 1980, 45,467 in 1990, and 65,838 in 1994. The ages of divorced couples range from the 20s to the 60s.

Summary

The characteristics of the movement in Korean women's population are the advance of age according to the continuous low level of birth rate; decrease in that part of the population capable of conception; increase of the young, unmarried population; and increase of divorce.

Participation in Economic Activities

Korea's economically active population, the country's total labor power, has increased from 20,326 in 1993 to 57,200 (2.9%) in 1994, reaching 473,400 (3.3%) in 1995. The labor market has been consistently expanding. When focusing on the increase of the population of men and women separately, between 1989 and 1994, the economically active population of men showed an increase from 9,617,000 to 12,167,000 (26%), while the population of women showed an increase at a higher rate, from 5,975,000 to 8,159,000 (36%).

This increase reflects women's desire to participate in economic activities and a growing number of opportunities for working women. This change can be viewed in four ways:

1. In the course of establishing and enacting an employment law giving equality to both sexes, the society's public opinion has changed to affirm women's economic activities.
2. Increased production of durable goods and consumption, as well as the growing wish for additional income, has motivated women to take part in society's activities.
3. A declining birth rate, lessening middle-age women's concerns about breast feeding, and an increasing supply of household appliances, simplifying household labor, have provided women more time to participate in the labor market.
4. The expanding industrial structure has opened a new field of industry where genuine labor, particularly labor for married women, is a necessity.

The *1993 Yearbook of Labor Statistics* shows that women of developed countries rate high in labor participation. For 1992, Korea's women's economic activity participation rate was 47.3%; Japan's, 50.7%; the United States', 56%; and England's, 51.7%. The participation of women ages 15 to 64, ages when practical activities are possible, was somewhat different. Korea showed an average rate of 50.2%, compared to Japan's 58.3%, the United States' 67%, and England's 51.7%. These figures show that women of developed countries have a higher labor participation rate than do women of Korea.

HEALTH ISSUES

Drinking

Following the 1980s' consumptive culture, Korean women have gradually increased their consumption of alcohol. According to the 1992 survey of national health and health awareness conducted by the Health Society Research Center, the rate of women who do not drink (67%) exceeds that of men (15.3%). And the rate of men who drink daily (9.9%) exceeds that of women (0.8%). This rate of daily drinkers has increased together with the increase of the average life span, reaching 13% among those ages 50 to 59. Men in this age bracket show a rate of 23.8%, also exceeding the women's rate of 1.9%.

Smoking

Smoking is one of today's most pressing health issues. Eighty-five percent of lung cancer is caused by smoking, and the possibility of smokers dying of lung cancer is 10 times greater than that of nonsmokers. Smoking constitutes 50% to 70% of larynx cancer, 50% of esophagus cancer, and 30% to 40% of bladder cancer.

Smokers are apt to be affected approximately 23% more easily than nonsmokers. Then there is the problem of nonsmokers who suffer physical harm indirectly caused by "secondhand" smoke.

When a young woman smokes, it not only harms her health for a long period, but also results in direct harmful effects to her generative functions and the child's health. When a pregnant woman smokes, it causes an increased danger to her health, and may cause a spontaneous abortion or premature birth. Smoking during pregnancy also gives rise to the birth of underweight babies.

Fortunately, the percentage of smokers in Korea is declining. The rate of men who smoke decreased from 73.2% in 1992 to 73% in 1995, and the rate of women smokers decreased from 6.1% to 6% in the same years.

Drug Abuse

The abuse of drugs is directly related to women's health. Drugs taken during pregnancy can cause great harm to the child, such as congenital malformation, abortion, and stillbirth. The legal usage of drugs also can affect a person's health and create serious problems.

However, the actual state of intoxicating and habitual drug abuse is difficult to ascertain. Once a person becomes addicted, programs for treatment and recovery do not have much effect on the addiction; thus, the need and demand for drugs continue to intensify.

A study of 1,408 adults in Seoul (49.2% women, 50.8% men) showed the number of people who had experience with drugs was 157, a rate of 11.1%. These people were again divided into those who used antihypnotic or hypnotic drugs (8.7%), marijuana (1.4%), organic compounds (1.1%), cocaine (0.8%), opium (0.2%), and Philopon (0.2%).

Participants in their 20s (16.3%) rated highest in drug use, followed by those in their 30s (10.5%), 40s (6.6%), and 50s (5.5%). In addition, 15% of unmarried singles were shown to have taken drugs, confirming the rapid spread of drug abuse among young people.

Nutrition

Nutrition is important to the maintenance and improvement of women's health. The recommended nutrient allowances are set in accordance with age, gender, weight, height, and amount of activity.

Females ages 10 to 12, though exceeding males in height and weight, receive less than the recommended energy allowances per day. This tends to be true of every age group. For example, males and females show similar differences in recommended protein allowances. Also, the recommended allowances of calcium is approximately the same in males and females. Women have a higher risk of osteoporosis as they reach the stage of menopause. This can be prevented by increased intake of calcium. Bone density increases consistently until age 35, then declines greatly during the following 6 to 10 years.

Recommended nutrient allowances have more importance than merely providing the average amount of nutrition needed for a person each day. The differences in amount, as shown in the recommended allowances, can also be reflected in the practical amount of intake. In a country like Korea, affected deeply by the patriarchal Confucianism culture, guidelines for women's nutrition intake has in many cases been conducted by men. Therefore, a detailed examination into the differences between males and females also must be considered.

The 1992 national nutrition examination survey, conducted by the Health and Society Ministry (1992), showed 4.9% of women with Body Mass Index (BMI) 15 and under, a rate higher than that of men's. The body mass index is a comparative percentage of weight and height, and BMI

15 indicates obesity. In rural regions, women's Body Nutrition Insufficiency Index (BNII) rate (5.0%) is higher than men's (3.7%), illustrating the seriousness of malnutrition among women in rural regions. But women's BMI exceeds men's both in the city and rural regions; clearly women show an imbalance in the amount of nutrition they absorb. However, estimating the nutritive conditions solely by means of BMI is an issue that must be reevaluated.

OTHER HEALTH ISSUES

Social factors have negatively affected Korean women's health. The discriminative social system negatively impacts women's economic and social capacities as well as their accessibility to healthcare services. Women make up nearly half (48%) of the economically active population. Such women suffer from pressures caused by double role play. They are exposed not only to poor labor conditions but also to the stress of being both mother at home and active participant in the workforce.

Due to an economy-centered development policy, the past 40 years of industrialization in Korean society have created neglected health conditions for women. As a result, there are increased mortality and cancer rates and incidences of artificial abortion, AIDS, and diseases of the genitourinary, mental disorders, suicide, and violence among women.

Incidence Rate of Diseases—Acute and Chronic

The following statistics were formulated from a 1993 survey conducted by the Korean Institute of Health and Social Affairs. For every 1,000 persons, women showed a higher incidence rate of acute diseases (209.4) as compared to men (171.9). Women also showed a higher rate than men for chronic diseases (320.8 versus 222.9). Women showed a higher rate (37.5) in acute diseases and also a higher rate (97.9) in chronic diseases. Among the 17 divisions of diseases, women show a higher incidence rate of acute diseases in 15 items, not including infections, parasitic diseases, injury, and poisoning. In chronic diseases, women show a higher incidence rate in 13 items, excluding infections and parasitic diseases, but including diseases of the respiratory area and of the skin. To make the comparison between the two sexes possible, diseases of genitourinary, exclusively in women, are combined in this item.

In the diseases of genitourinary, the incidence rate of acute diseases in women is 7.3–12.2 times that of men (0.6). In injury and poisoning, mental disorder, and disease of the circulatory system, women show 1.9, 1.8, and 1.8 times, respectively, the amount shown in men. In chronic diseases, women show a higher incidence rate—2.34 times the amount in signs and ill-defined conditions, 2.11 times the amount in diseases of the musculoskeletal, 1.7 times in diseases of the nervous system, 1.7 times in diseases of the circulatory system, and 1.6 times in mental disorders. Overall, women suffer more pains from chronic diseases than men. Since diseases of the musculoskeletal system; circulatory system; endocrine, nutritional, and metabolic systems; and nervous system show a sudden rise after the age of 50, prevention plans should be started from age 20 and upward.

Incidence of Cancer

Cancers, exclusively concerning women, are cervical cancer, breast cancer, and tumors of the ovaries. When the area of cancer development is compared in its frequency in both sexes (Table 4.1), one can find a difference in pattern between the two.

Table 4.1   Frequency of Cancer

	Male			Female		
Rank	Type	Number of Cases	%	Type	Number of Cases	%
1	Stomach	8,246	(28.3)	Cervix	4,975	(22.0)
2	Lung	4,597	(15.7)	Stomach	4,017	(17.9)
3	Liver	4,380	(15.0)	Breast	571	(11.4)
4	Large intestine	2,056	(7.1)	Large intestine	1,637	(7.5)
5	Esophagus	954	(3.3)	Lung	1,262	(5.3)
6	Bladder	882	(3.0)	Liver	1,192	(5.3)
7	Gall bladder	830	(2.9)	Thymid	1,174	(5.2)
8	Hematopoietic	794	(2.7)	Gall bladder	655	(2.9)
9	Larynx	653	(2.2)	Ovary	647	(2.9)

Source: National Statistical Office (1996).

Women show the highest frequency of cancer development in the cervix (22.0%), followed by the stomach (17.9%) and breast (11.4%). Men show the highest frequency of cancer in the stomach, lung, and liver. The percentage rate that breast cancer constituted on the national rate for women was 8.9% in the 1980s; it abruptly increased to 11.4% in 1993. Some of the risk factors that make woman more prone to breast cancer are family history, heredity, dietary patterns (high calorie intake, high fat content in diets), obesity, and use of birth control pills. Tumors of the ovaries constituted 2.9%.

The occurrence rate of cancer is higher in females between the ages of 30 and 40, but is higher in men over 50. Among male patients, 6.5% are in their 30s and 13.4% are in their 40s. But in female patients, 15.4% are in their 30s and 18.8% are in their 40s. Until the age of 40, there are more female cancer patients than male cancer patients. A large amount of information concerning the prevention of uterocervical cancer through pap smear tests has been delivered. But more information should be given on the prevention of breast cancer through self-testing or tests using mammography.

Induced Abortion

Except in special circumstances, induced abortion is illegal in Korea. Nevertheless, the rate of induced abortions is very high.

The number of induced abortions increased to 1979, and decreased the following years before increasing in 1991. Although there is an increase in the rate of women using contraception, the rate of induced abortions has not decreased. The Korea Institute of Health and Social Affairs reported that in 1993, 70% of the women in the age group of 20–24 who had induced abortions, were single. Until 1979, the age group of 30–39 showed a high rate of induced abortions (156), but the rate later dropped in large degrees to 25 in 1993. Induced abortions of the 1970s were carried out as a part of family planning policy. (For successful family planning, appropriate numbers of children were delivered.) In cases where pregnancies had to be terminated, permanent contraceptive surgery was conducted. The cities show higher rates of induced abortion in all age groups and especially in the age group of 20–29. The total number of induced abortion cases reached an estimated 490,000 in the year 1993. Another survey shows that 33% of all cases of induced abortion were conducted on single women.

The reason for the increase of induced abortions in younger age groups can be explained by the change in sexual awareness and culture. Induced abortions not only affect maternal health, but also affect the overall health of women. Of the married women who had induced abortions in 1988, 17% experienced side effects such as hemorrhage, lumbago, and weakness. The mortality rate was high.

Induced abortions are done in cases mainly of unwanted pregnancies, so the practice of contraception should reduce the induced abortion incidence rate.

HIV/AIDS and Other Sexually Transmitted Diseases

The total number of Korean HIV positive patients as of February 1996 was 608, 75 of whom were women (14.9%). Among HIV/AIDS patients, the age group of 21 to 31 makes up 505. (See Table 4.2.)

The survey data for the incidence rate of sexually transmitted diseases are limited. "The Study of Health Insurance Policy" conducted by the Korea Institute of Health and Social Affairs in 1990 surveyed those who used medical facilities authorized for health insurance of sexually transmitted diseases. The subjects of this study (617 individuals: 335 general patients and 282 supervised patients) were 87.2% (292 individuals) male. Of those women supervised patients, 95% were being treated for sexually transmitted diseases.

In these supervised patients, the number of cases showed gonorrhea as the most frequent, followed by gonococcal urethritis, and syphilis. Syphilis, known to be the most fatal among the sexually transmitted diseases, had a relatively high percentage of 11.7%.

Table 4.2 Number of Cases of HIV Infection and Death Cases in 1985–1989, 1990–1996 (in Persons)

	1989	1990	1991	1992	1993	1994	1995	1996	Total	Male	Female
Total	73	44	42	76	78	90	108	87	607	533	75
	5	2	1	2	6	11	14	22	63	38	25
	28	13	9	14	9	13	13	5	104	91	13
	45	41	33	62	69	17	95	82	503		

Source: Ministry of Health and Welfare, News Report (1996).

The patriarchal culture of Korea emphasized chastity in women while allowing freer sexual practices for men. As a result, men brought the risk of sexually transmitted disease to their spouses or partners.

Mental Disorders and Suicide Rate

In Korea, there are more women with mental disorders than men. There are 3 women with mental disorders for every hundred, which amounts to 33.5% of the total number of mental disorder patients. This means that among the mental disorder patients two-thirds are women, twice the number of male patients. Also, the number of women with Depression is twice that of men, with many of them diagnosed as neurotic, suffering from anxiety (fear of predicted loss).

Neuroses and Depression may be consequences of a male-centered culture. Women are treated differently, and their role brings about conflict. Discrimination between sexes exists in various situations, aggravating mental problems and making women feel incapable of finding solutions. Women's mental health is greatly influenced by the social attitudes toward married/single women; childless women; mothers; poor, abused, and divorced women; women of minority groups; widows; old women; and passionate women.

Other causes of Depression in women include sterility, unhappy marriages, physical and sexual abuse, poverty, and loneliness in old age. Full-time mothers, when pregnant, show more signs of Depression than women with jobs.

There has been an analysis of the language used by Asian/Pacific women to find out why they experience more psychological pain than men. The results show the reasons to be (a) stress and tension from additional pressure from labor, (b) institutionalized sex roles and expectancy, and (c) increased awareness of rights and choices which influences family and marital relationship adaptability.

The morbidity rate of mental disorder in women is higher in all age groups except that of 0 to 9. Women show twice the rate of incidence between ages 20 and 69, when women are most active in sexual and familial relationships. They show the highest rate of incidence between 30 and 59, when the roles of mother in pregnancy and childcare are concentrated.

Suicide attempts are higher in women. The reasons for suicide in women are shown to be family problems, especially physical and psychological abuse from husbands, and legal problems concerning pregnancy outside of marriage or divorce (condemned by Korean society). Women suffer mental and psychological pressures from socially and culturally discriminative situations.

MORTALITY RATE

It is important to see that diseases of the circulatory system comprise the number-one cause of death in Korean men and women. But the second and third leading causes differ between the two sexes. The second leading cause for men is neoplasms and the third, injury and poisoning, while women have signs and ill-defined conditions as second, and neoplasms for the third leading causes of death. This pattern has not changed over time. Due to the mainly negative taboos in Korean culture concerning women, not much data on women is available. This serves as an impediment to the promotion of women's health and dissemination of information and preparation of preventive alternatives.

The rate of institutionalized childbirth was already 97% in the year 1987 and increased to 99.1% from 1987 to 1991. Nevertheless, the infant and maternal mortality rate is still high. The infant mortality rate decreased from 60% in 1960 to 1.6% in 1993, but the numbers of the population increased from 25 million to 44 million. Also the number of women who are capable of pregnancy increased from 5.85 million to 12.7 million. Because of these reasons, the number of newborn babies has not altered much. In recent years, this number was about 670,000 annually.

Infant and maternal mortality rates, used as an international index of maternal health, are decreasing in Korea. Infant mortality is 12.8 for every 1,000 newly born babies and maternal mortality is 14 for every 10 mothers. When this is applied to an annual total number of newborn babies (670,000), 200 mothers die yearly due to childbirth; direct obstetrical causes account for only 85 cases. When maternal mortality rate is compared with the international data of 1991 (13.7 per 100,000 women in Korea) shows that Korea is 5 times higher than the lowest, which is Singapore, with 2.1 per 100,000 women. The other countries are also less than 10, so it can be said that Korea's maternal mortality rate is quite high. Since the rate can be easily lowered with preventive measures, medical personnel should be responsible for finding risk factors in pregnant women before and after delivery. They should also avoid dangerous surgical operations during delivery and improve medical practice so as to decrease maternal mortality. This would be more effective if nurses would constantly look for and be aware of abuse of medical treatment.

MEDICAL SERVICES

In the previous sections, the demographical characteristics and actual conditions of factors related to health in women were discussed. Women were, in general, higher in the incidence rate for both acute and chronic diseases than men and had a higher rate of visitation to hospitals. Because the position of women in the family and society is low, they are not given enough support. For example, when women are diagnosed with the same diseases as men, they show a higher rate of visitation. But the rate of hospitalization for women is lower than men; and when they are indeed hospitalized, they are not retained for a sufficient amount of time. In cases where women are hospitalized for complications due to pregnancy, child delivery, and puerperal diseases, their hospital stays are shorter than when they have other diseases.

The rate of women in the health field profession is highest in nurses and maternity nurses. In 1995, 58.4% of the licensed pharmacists were female; 17.8% of those were doctors; 20.2%, dentists; and 8.1%, doctors of Chinese medicine.

SUGGESTIONS FOR THE FUTURE

The health conditions of Korean women and other related facts have been examined and discussed. Some suggestions regarding these topics include:

1. Health centers managed by nurses should be constructed in every community. They should be accessible to women and should also promote easy diffusion of information on female health education. These health centers should alleviate impediments in the use of female health services and also plan and operate health programs that the community needs.
2. The decision process of the health policy for women should be related to feminist groups and their suggestions should be efficiently reflected to improve women's health rights. There should also be

stronger laws and changes in the government to guarantee necessary changes in the governmental system, and a guarantee of necessary conditions for women to use their rights.

3. Women with HIV should be protected and policies and programs for them should be developed to guarantee their participation. Special educational programs should be utilized and supported.

4. Studies related to women's health should be encouraged, and the government should support anti-breast cancer movements and non-smokers' movements.

REFERENCES

Chang, P. (1996a). *The rise of women's education against the Korean patriarching.* Seoul: Asian Center for Woman's Studies, Ewha Womans University.

Chang, P. (1996b). *Woman, sex, health.* Seoul: Asia Women's Center.

Chang, Y. S. (1997). *Population and policy development public welfare Forcus, 4.* Seoul: The Research Center for Korea Public Health and Social.

ILO Year Book of Lavor Statistics. (1991, 1995).

Kane, P. (1994). *Women's health from womb to tomb.* London: St. Martin's Press.

Korca Daily News Paper. (1995).

National Statistical Office. (1996). Major Indication in OECD.

Raunsley, M. (1996). *Phenomenon of related health in women (presentation): Expanding the research agenda.*

Robert, H. (1992). *Women's health matters.* New York: Routledge.

Shin, K. R. (1997). A study on the health status of adult women in island. *The Journal of Korea Adult Nursing Academic Society.*

Sterm, P. (1996). *Conceptualizing women's health: Discovering the dimensions* (presentation). Seoul: Ewha Woman's University, College of Nursing Science.

The Fourth World Women's Conference in Beijing. (1995). *Action principles.* Seoul: The Korea Women's Development Center.

World Health Organization. (1984). *World Statistics Annual.*

World Health Organization. (1988). "Health for all" series #1. Geneva, Switzerland: Author.

World Health Organization Alma-Ata. (1978). *Primary health care.* Geneva, Switzerland: Author.

Yearbook of Health and Social Statistics. (1994). *Ministry of health and social affairs.* Republic of Korea.

CHAPTER FIVE

Elderly Filipino Women's Adjustment to Widowhood: Implications for Health and Well-Being

Geraldine Valencia-Go, PhD, RN, CS

Widowhood begins with the death of a spouse. It affects more women then men because women tend to marry older men and have longer life spans (Brubaker, 1985; Eliopoulos, 1997). Death can occur unexpectantly at a time of apparent good health, or after much anticipation, as in the case of degenerative or terminal illnesses (Brubaker, 1985). Whatever the circumstances surrounding the death of one's spouse, the partner left behind experiences grief, loss, and mourning. There is a concurrent loss of many roles, particularly those directly related to the deceased spouse (Wakin, 1980). For widowed women, the loss of a spouse also can mean losing an "accustomed level of living" (Heinemann, 1982, p. 20), a result of reduced income. The unemployed widowed woman can experience loss of benefits tied with her husband's employment as well (Eliopoulos, 1997). Interactions with kin and friends can decline or be lost as "life style differences become apparent and result in divergent interests, experiences, and values" (Heinemann, 1982, p. 20). Loss of self-esteem and self-worth can cause a widowed woman to lose her identity as she attempts to fill the roles of the deceased spouse. Therefore, widowed women face a realm of potential financial, legal, and social problems.

Widowed women experience a host of grief symptoms classified as (a) affective, (b) behavioral manifestations, (c) attitude toward self and the deceased, (d) cognitive impairment, and (e) physiological changes and bodily complaints (Stroebe & Stroebe, 1987). Multiple losses coupled with the

58

range of grief symptoms leave the widowed woman physically and mentally vulnerable.

CULTURAL ASPECTS OF WIDOWHOOD

A woman's adjustment to widowhood is a developmental task of successful aging (Havighurst, 1972). For Filipino women, whose experiences are addressed in this chapter, widowhood represents not only a major loss of a relationship, but also because of voluntary immigration, it represents a loss of one's native land, culture, friends, and an array of supportive relationships.

In order to understand Filipino women's responses to widowhood, it is essential to note that their cultural heritage consists primarily of Chinese, Hispanic, and Malayan origins. From this heritage, cultural customs and mores have guided Filipino women in many aspects of their daily lives. With the loss of a spouse, these women are confronted with the demands and expectations of the loss, and their responses are largely guided by the influence of Chinese culture.

In the traditional Chinese culture, widowhood generally means a life of misery for the woman. Because she and her children are considered the property of her in-laws, she cannot remarry freely. Furthermore, Chinese men consider her a "second class article" (Yang, 1959, p. 111); therefore her opportunities are truly limited. The woman who chooses to leave her children with in-laws faces the dilemma of her children's potential abuse and unfair allotments of her dead husband's assets and properties. She herself may suffer abuse and humiliation from her in-laws, who later on may require her to care for them in their old age (Lang, 1946). If she does remarry, her children, regarded as aliens in her new husband's community, face the same ill treatment, discrimination, and exclusion from her new husband's family. With this cultural heritage, what is a widowed Filipino woman to do?

WIDOWED FILIPINO WOMEN IMMIGRANTS

Valencia-Go (1989) conducted a qualitative study of 14 widowed Filipino women who immigrated to the United States. One purpose of this study was to discover the impact of the widowhood experience in later life events such as immigration.

Among these women, the youngest was 68, the oldest 86. The woman longest widowed lost her husband 45 years previous; the most recently widowed woman lost her husband just 2 years before the study. Eight of the women now have become American citizens, and six have become permanent residents. The earliest immigrant came in 1974; the most recent arrival came in 1987. Ten of these women live with their daughters and their families, and two live with sons and their children. The remaining two widows are homeowners, and their children rent living quarters from them (Valencia-Go, 1989).

Only two women maintained employment outside the home. The other twelve cared for preschool and school-age children, and also were responsible for such household chores as cooking and washing—tasks that alleviated the burdens of women who maintained full-time careers. Only three women had earned college degrees; the rest ended their formal education in the fourth through seventh grades (Valencia-Go, 1989).

GRIEF AND THE WIDOWHOOD EXPERIENCE

Arnold (1996), in her reformulation of grief, believes that in grieving "one integrates loss and maintain's one's connectedness to the lost person or object and learns to live without" (p. 777). Consistent with this statement, Valencia-Go's study discovered that earlier adjustments and adaptations to widowhood provided a Filipino woman with necessary coping mechanisms and strategies to integrate positively into a new culture, nurture family relationships, and optimize health and well-being. In this study, the grounded theory methodology formulated by Glaser and Strauss (1967) was used. Through in-depth interviews and analyses of the data, several themes were derived. These themes are like threads woven to create a cohesive whole that is the widowed woman's experience, and they include women's perceptions of their spouse, the grief process, and their current perspectives on the widowhood experience.

Women's Perceptions of Their Spouse

When asked to describe their husband, widowed women described individuals focused on their roles and responsibilities in the family. This emphasis on familial roles reflected the women's strong cultural orientation regarding the position of Filipino men (Vreeland, Hurwitz, Jurst, Moeller, & Shinn, 1976). One woman said:

My husband was a very hard-working man. He even went to the rice fields on Sundays. When I challenged this behavior, I got this answer, "Why don't we have to eat on Sundays?"

All but two women said their husbands were considerate, loving, and thoughtful. One woman explained:

My husband was very loving and protective of me. He was kind and gentle. He would make me laugh whenever he saw me in a bad mood.

Another woman, who was the major breadwinner in her marriage, believed that the role reversal was accepted by both her and her husband. She explained:

We treated each other as individuals. I was excellent at business and management, whereas my husband excelled at cooking and keeping the house clean and neat. He always waited for me and always had a nice dinner prepared.

In summary, Filipino women's behavioral expressions of their grief were consistent with findings from other studies on widowhood. Behavioral expressions included weeping for the spouse, yearning for his presence, and remembering him fondly (Thompson, Thompson, Futterman, Gilewski, & Peterson, 1991).

The Grief Process

The women described their behaviors, feelings, and thoughts; their subsequent adjustments; and the support they received. Disbelief and shock were the primary reactions during the first few weeks following the spouse's death. They all experienced weeks or months of restlessness, depression with long periods of weeping, lack of appetite, and insomnia. Sanders (1992) described many of the same behaviors and feelings in her work with grief and learning how to survive it. She heard statements like those that follow:

I can't remember clearly what I did then. I stayed home most of the time. I was like "mindless" and thought often of my husband and how I will raise my children without him. I could not listen to what other people were saying. I kept on crying and crying. I felt lonely and depressed. Every time I thought about him, I would break into tears.

Acceptance and realization of the husband's death came within days for some, months and years for others. If the husband's death was due to illness, women were angry and blamed doctors, labeling them incompetent. The women also wondered whether they did everything possible to save their spouse. With acceptance and realization, the women began to think about their future and the children still to rear.

All of the women had supportive family and friends who took over some of their husband's roles. Those women with careers outside the home were able to continue working. In cases where the now deceased husband had been a business owner, within a year most of the widowed women gained full control of the business. And those who were previously homemakers were successful in establishing some type of enterprise. The courage and strength of these women can be recognized in this woman's statement:

> *I had to get hold of myself and assume the roles of my husband. There were the rice fields and all the crops we sold. I had to do all that and my children to think about.*

Support women received from family and friends was critical for adjustment and reintegration into their communities as widowed women. One woman perceived her oldest son's support during her time of grief as most important. She would talk to him about his father and often sought answers to her questions:

> *Why do I have to suffer like this? I asked him. He said, "God chooses only those who have the strength and courage and He knows that you can take it." I really could not handle it, but had to since Mike (the son) and everyone felt I could.*

Other family members such as adult children contributed financially and assumed the time-consuming task of caring for younger siblings.

All the women in the study were able to fulfill their tasks and parental roles with the help of children, other family members, and friends. Additionally, the women believed they were able to handle their new roles because of self-determination and strength. These women's perceived strength as a result of widowhood was validated in a more recent study on widowhood and depression (see Umberson, Wortman, & Kessler, 1992).

This successful resolution of grief and positive adjustment facilitated an optimistic and positive anticipation of the future.

Women's Perspectives on Widowhood

The women's feelings and views regarding widowhood were partly comprised of rewards; successes, particularly independence; resources gained; regrets and other negative feelings.

For most of the women, the widowhood experience was felt to be a growth-enhancing process with many rewards and successes. They attributed these successes to inner strength giving them courage to face new situations. One woman commented:

> *If I was not widowed, I would not have learned to live with our tenants, the grass-roots level. There were all those poor around me, with almost nothing, yet they seem so content and happy. I saw that I had more than they, and I knew then that I would live.*

Another woman said:

> *I am able to work and get a paying job outside the home. I don't ask anyone to come with me when I look for work. I am very determined. I have to!*

All the women believed they gained an important asset—independence, which they defined as the ability to rely on oneself and make decisions. According to the women, independence means not having to rely on children, relatives, and friends for financial assistance. The women said the widowhood experience motivated them to "stand on their own feet." They realized that earlier attempts to fill the roles of their spouse facilitated their quests to succeed in any enterprise they undertook.

In spite of the women's positive outlook, negative aspects of the widowhood experience were emphasized. These negative aspects were accentuated by the aging process, current relationships with children, deteriorating health, and stresses of immigration. One Filipino woman commented:

> *My life is one big sacrifice and sadness. I had no luck because my husband died during our earlier years of marriage, and then I spent my whole life educating these five children by myself. I am very proud and happy that I have given them something. Perhaps, if I had not sacrificed, these five lives would not be what they are today. But now everyone has a family and I am really alone in my old age. I could have remarried but I don't think it would work. So, here I am.*

Another woman who took over the management of her husband's lumber business and reared nine children said:

> *When my husband died, I carried the business and I was able to pay my children's tuition and give them most of the things they wanted. I sent them to the schools of their choice. Now, I feel isolated and lonely. I only want some show of affection and concern from my children. They could at least ask me how I feel and spend a little time talking about my concerns.*

In general, the widowhood experience was considered with a mix of mostly positive and a few negative aspects. Since widowhood was perceived as the major change in their lives, the women capitalized on ensuing experiences and now use those to cope with current situations. One such situation is immigration, which in many respects represents loss.

GAINS FROM LOSSES: IMPLICATIONS FOR HEALTH AND WELL-BEING

The widowed Filipino women's successful resolution of grief and their emergence as individuals with new identities represented more than the achievement of a developmental task proposed by Havighurst (1972). The process of grieving, new roles, tasks, and adjustments had all been part of a larger adaptive task that ensured the integration of these widowed women into their families and society.

Lopata (1975) wrote that "American society is still socializing women to be wives and mothers and not to have alternate identities available at any stage of the life cycle" (p. 15). Filipino culture is still, to a large extent, very similar in its orientation in regard to the roles of women. Block, Davidson, and Grambs (1986) asserted that women by virtue of their longer life spans have many options. "They choose to focus more on themselves and less on responsibility toward others" (p. 76). For these Filipino women, their choices of lifestyle were guided by their sense of ethnicity and personal commitment to the role of mother. They had reconstructed their lives as single women and acquired new roles. Women's adjustment to widowhood was validated in Porter's (1994) study on widows living alone. Porter identified four major phenomena; they are "(a) making aloneness acceptable, (b) going my way, (c) reducing risks, and (d) sustaining myself" (p. 21).

Children and their well-being continue to be concerns of widowed Filipino women, who consider their children as main resources. These women exhibit commitment and competence in a "new social world that responds to them individually, not as former wives or widows" (Lopata, 1975, p. 53). As they continue to age in this culture—so different from their own, they consider themselves determined, intelligent, resourceful, and independent. They often look back at their many difficulties, but at the same time they are grateful for their rewards and successes. Thus, it can be said that these women are valuing widowhood as a positive experience.

Valencia-Go's (1989) study of widowed Filipino women showed that the experience of losing a spouse and the concomitant loss of roles and relationships were positive milestones in these women's lives. The shared experiences of these women are important contributions in the work of nurses and other healthcare professionals who work with individuals during the grieving period. Healthcare professionals know that following a loss, health can deteriorate when basic needs of food and sleep are neglected. Often family members and friends involved in other matters fail to see symptoms. Nurses and healthcare workers could work with a designated family member or even a close friend to provide oversight of the widowed person's physiological needs. Help with grocery shopping and food preparation not only addresses physiological needs but also provides social support to the bereaved person. Provisions for long-term monitoring, such as making healthcare appointments and accompanying women to them, are extremely helpful. Moreover, these women should be made aware of the increased risk for accidents during times of high levels of stress (Anderson & Dimond, 1995).

Depression in widowed persons has been researched extensively (Feinson, 1986; Gallagher, Breckenridge, Thompson, & Peterson, 1983; Zissok, Shuchter, & Lyons, 1987). Healthcare workers, family members, and friends should be aware that persistent depression is not a normal part of grieving, and they should facilitate care and treatment for the bereaved individual (Anderson & Dimond, 1995).

Social support and its importance in alleviating depression was documented earlier by Bowling (1988) and Cobb (1976). More recently, Kanacki, Jones, and Galbraith (1996) related higher levels of social support to lower depression scores for widowed men and women. Nurses and other healthcare workers should alert the widowed person's family and friends to signs of persistent depression and work with them in creating a circle of support. Referrals to groups and organizations are essential so that family members and friends have resources when they are unable to visit or otherwise spend time with the bereaved person.

As the community becomes an important healthcare resource, nurses and other healthcare workers should facilitate the organization of support groups. As neighborhoods and communities become more ethnically diverse, those organizing support groups need to consider specific cultural traditions that could enhance energy and interest critical in maintaining the viability of the group.

Widowed persons, such as this study's Filipino women, who successfully resolved their grief and gained from their many losses, can serve as positive role models for others. These women could share their unique way of coping and dealing with losses and pains. What a wonderful way to give to others, by sharing in the experience of gaining a new self after a loss.

REFERENCES

Anderson, K. L., & Dimond, M. F. (1995). The experience of bereavement in older adults. *Journal of Advanced Nursing, 22,* 308-315.

Arnold, J. (1996). Rethinking grief: Nursing implications for health promotion. *Home Healthcare Nurse, 14*(10), 777-783.

Block, M., Davidson, J. L., & Grambs, J. D. (1986). *Women over forty: Visions and reality.* New York: Springer.

Bowling, A. (1988). Who dies after widow(er)hood? A discriminant analysis. *Omega, 19,* 135-153.

Brubaker, T. (1985). *Later life families: Family studies series: I.* Beverly Hills, CA: Sage.

Cobb, S. (1976). Social support as a moderator of life stress. *Psychosomatic Medicine, 38,* 300-314.

Eliopoulos, C. (1997). *Gerontological nursing* (4th ed.). Philadelphia: Lippincott.

Feinson, M. C. (1986). Aging widows and widowers: Are there mental health differences? *International Journal of Aging and Development, 23,* 241-255.

Gallagher, D. E., Breckenridge, J. N., Thompson, L. W., & Peterson, J. A. (1983). Effects of bereavement on indicators of mental health in elderly widows and widowers. *Journal of Gerontology, 38,* 565-571.

Glaser, B. G., & Strauss, A. L. (1967). *The discovery of grounded theory.* Chicago: Aldine.

Havighurst, R. (1972). *Developmental tasks and education* (3rd ed.). New York: David McKay.

Heinemann, G. D. (1982, Summer). Why study widowed women: A rationale. *Women and Health, 7,* 17-29.

Kanacki, L. S., Jones, P. S., & Galbraith, M. E. (1996, February). Social support and depression in widows and widowers. *Journal of Gerontological Nursing, 39-45.*

Lang, O. (1946). *Chinese family and society.* New Haven, CT: Yale University Press.

Lopata, H. Z. (1975). On widowhood: Grief, work and identity reconstruction. *Journal of Geriatric Psychiatry, 31,* 41-55.

Porter, E. J. (1994). Older widows' experience of living alone. *Image: Journal of Nursing Scholarship, 26*(1), 19-24.

Sanders, C. M. (1992). *Surviving grief and learning to live again.* New York: Wiley.

Stroebe, W., & Stroebe, M. S. (1987). *Bereavement and health: The psychological and physical consequences of partner loss.* New York: Cambridge University Press.

Thompson, L. W., Thompson, D. G., Futterman, A., Gilewski, M. J., & Peterson, J. (1991). The effects of late-life spousal bereavement over a 30-month interval. *Psychology and Aging, 6*(3), 434-441.

Umberson, D., Wortman, C. B., & Kessler, M. C. (1992). Widowhood and depression: Explaining long-term gender differences in vulnerability. *Journal of Health and Social Behavior, 33,* 10-24.

Valencia-Go, G. (1989). Integrative aging in widowed immigrant Filipinas: A grounded theory study. *Dissertation Abstracts International.* p. 1-300. (University Microfilms No. 8923910).

Vreeland, N., Hurwitz, G. B., Jurst, P., Moeller, P. W., & Shinn, R. S. (1976). *Area handbook for the Philippines* (2nd ed.) (DA PAM 550-72). Washington, DC: U.S. Government Printing Office.

Wakin, E. (1980). Living as a widow: Only the name's the same. In M. M. Fuller & C. A. Martin (Eds.), *The older woman: Lavender rose or gray panther* (pp. 151-157). Springfield, IL: Thomas.

Yang, C. K. (1959). *The Chinese family in the Communist Revolution.* Cambridge Center for International Studies: Massachusetts Institute of Technology.

Zissok, S., Schuchter, S. R., & Lyons, L. E. (1987). Predictors of psychological reactions during the early stages of widowhood. *Psychiatric Clinics of North America, 10,* 355-368.

CHAPTER SIX

Healthcare Problems Among Filipinos in Hawaii with a Focus on the Filipino Elderly

Clementina D. Ceria, PhD, RN

Yoshiko Shimamoto, PhD, RN

*F*ilipinos comprise the third largest Asian American group, representing 20.6% of the Asian population (U.S. Department of Commerce, Bureau of Census, 1993a). Only the Japanese and Chinese Americans outnumber the Filipinos. In the United States, Filipinos number 1,406,770 (San Buanaventura, 1995). They live in the West (52.4%), Northeast (27%), South (12.4%), and Midwest (8.1%) (U.S. Department of Commerce, Bureau of Census, 1993b).

There are 168,862 Filipinos living in Hawaii, making them the third largest ethnic group in the state (Weygan-Hildebrand, 1995). The Hawaii Sugar Planters Association imported Filipino laborers under a contract system that was regulated by a 1915 Act. Contracts guaranteed a return passage to the Philippines after three years in Hawaii. Most Filipinos were recruited from the Visayan tribes and districts of Ilocos Norte and Ilocos Sur. These early immigrants suffered acute sociopsychological problems from being separated from their families, causing subsequent social problems in their later years. In 1965 the immigration law put professional skills on an equal footing with national origin for immigrant entry. This attracted immigrants who were educated and possessed skills that were in demand. In 1974, 32,857 Filipinos immigrated to the United States. A large proportion worked in medical occupations in the northeastern, north central, southern, and western portions of the United States. The most recent immigrants to Hawaii are World War II Filipino-American veterans who were compensated for their war efforts with American citizenship (Weygan-Hildebrand, 1995).

THE PHILIPPINES

The Philippines is a country of contrasts with the highest level of civilization existing alongside primitive peoples. It includes 7,083 islands covering 114,000 square miles. A population of 35 million is divided into three geographical areas: the large northern island of Luzon, home to Manila and the adjacent islands of Mindoro and Palawan; the central group of the Visayas; and Mindanao, the largest and southernmost island of the Philippines. There are 87 dialects and 8 major languages, although Tagalog or Philipino is the national language and English, which is taught after the third grade, is unofficially the national language.

History

The Philippines was named for Don Felipe II of Spain after it was discovered in 1521 by Magellan. During three centuries of Spanish rule, the Filipinos developed a colonial mentality. Americans who arrived later contributed to this low self-esteem of the natives. However, the true rulers of the Philippines are Spanish-Filipino *mestizo* families (about 400 in number) interested in retaining great power and wealth (Jones, 1974).

Cultural Values and Beliefs

The four primary rules in traditional Filipino culture were (a) authority of male members, (b) seniority of age, (c) obedience of youth, and (d) collective responsibility. Based on strong family ties, children looked to parents for support up to the age of maturity. Parents took good care of their children, believing they were their old-age pensions (Lasker, 1940).

Filipino parents reared their children according to certain behavioral guidelines and value systems. The following behavioral expectations suggested by these operational procedures governed the lives of Filipinos (Zamora, 1967):

Amor propio was a sense of self-esteem or an exaggerated sense of self-worth. It was the need of the Filipino to be treated as a person. Filipinos were defensive toward any negative remarks, accounting for their extreme sensitivity.

Hiya was a form of self-depreciation and shame. The most important values were concern for the family as a group and respect for older Filipinos. Competition was frowned upon, yet one must rise above one's peers. Any wrong deed was a reflection on the group.

Pakikisama was a means of enforcing smooth interpersonal relationships even if it involved conceding to others' wishes. Mediators were used to bring about the least amount of confrontation and to minimize the possibility of shaming someone or having him or her "lose face." Direct confrontation, disagreement, and criticism were avoided.

Utang na loob involved reciprocal obligations that wove participants into a fabric of social alliances. It involved a give-and-take and provided a sense of social security, a certain perception of the world. "When you invest something, you also can expect something in return." This value of obligation was the foundation that maintained the closeness of the kinship system of the Philippines.

Bahala Na meant leaving things to fate or God. The Filipino was a fatalist, believing he had little or not control over his destiny and that good fortune was simply good luck.

The Malayan influence in the elderly Filipino accounted for the persistence of superstition, animism, belief in magic, fatalism, and group affinity. Filipinos believed in life after death, when the soul travels to another world to receive its due reward or punishment. The body was kept for a considerable period of time, and the spirits of the dead were addressed repeatedly. During the sixteen century, the Spaniards converted most Filipinos to Catholicism (Zaide, 1937). Therefore, Filipinos paid homage to the dead on November 1 by visiting their graves. But ancestor worship prevailed and it remained important to be on satisfactory terms with the souls of the dead. Some believed that these souls interacted with the living who had debts to pay, coercing them into settlement by plaguing them with sickness. The living then had to make sacrifices (Kroeber, 1928). The supernatural being called *anito,* a generic term in Tagalog, included gods, evil spirits, and souls of dead human beings. The Filipino feared *anito* and projected into the spirit world the same desires and passions which existed on earth. The spirits which belonged to their ancestors were good and those which belonged to their enemies were bad. To placate their wrath sacrifices often had to be offered.

Specific beliefs and acts varied among the ethnic groups, but Filipinos generally believed that medicine was influenced by magic, witchcraft, and sorcery. Medicinal substances were believed to operate magically rather than pharmaceutically (Kroeber, 1928), and ceremonies were designed to cure illness. There was a distinct ritual for each recognized disease or type of disease believed to have been caused by a particular class of spirits (Kroeber, 1928). Some superstitions were related to causes of illnesses. For example, if one dumps dirt or builds a fire on top of a mound, it will irk the *nuno sa punso* who lives there and cause the offender to become sick. If a young person wears a jacket reserved for the elderly Filipino, he or she will become ill. There was widespread belief in the *aswang,* which assumed the form of a dog, cat, or bird and ate human flesh; and in the *mangkukulam,* which caused people to get sick or die by pricking a toy with his magic pin (Zaide, 1937). Charms and amulets such as the *anting-anting,* which was a universal amulet, were popular.

Many superstitions remain today; for example, when a young girl sings before a stove or fire she will marry an old widower. And to play with your food could cause a stomachache (Ledesma, 1976). According to outreach workers, backwoods medical practitioners known as *arbularyos* (Zabilka, 1970) are not currently in practice, but *hilots,* who heal by massage using warm coconut oil and ginger, are in the contemporary Filipino community.

SEARCH STRATEGY

An extensive life span search was done through Medline, Hawaii Library System, Hawaii Medical Library, and Hawaii Pacific Index using terms such as *Filipino, Hawaii, health, problems,* and *diseases.* This search revealed just eight sources of information. Cultural beliefs and practices of the child rearing period among Filipino families living in Hawaii was written in 1954; an article on the incidence of sudden death of Filipino men in Hawaii, in 1964. Ethnicity and health in Hawaii and cardiovascular disease mortality among Filipinos were addressed in 1978. Two sources written in 1994 included a thesis on the cardiovascular disease risk in young Filipino women and a research report on peak bone mass of women living in Hawaii, which sampled Filipino women. In 1995, there was a study done on bone mineral content including Filipino children and an overview of the Filipinos living in Hawaii. Much of the literature dating from the 1920s to 1996 was about Filipino immigration (in the early 1900s and after 1965) to the United States, specifically to

Hawaii and California; Filipino adaptation to the United States—their struggles and everyday life in sugar cane plantation camps; and the formation of Filipino labor unions in Hawaii.

Because the available literature was so limited, the search was further specified to *Filipino* and *Hawaii* and *children* and *health* and *problem*. And an additional search was conducted using the same terms but for the substitution of *adolescent* for *children*. Neither search revealed relevant literature.

Therefore, the focus of this chapter is on the health problems of Filipinos as discussed by the literature obtained during the initial search.

HEALTH PROBLEMS

Chronic Diseases

The Research and Statistics Office of the Hawaii State Department of Health conducted a study to examine certain conditions and events among the various ethnic groups living in Hawaii. The study was based on a sample of 12,129 households with 40,193 persons. The conditions and events examined included (a) one or more chronic conditions experienced during the previous year, (b) one or more days of bed rest resulting from a chronic illness, (c) one or more nights of hospital inpatient care resulting from a chronic illness or pregnancy, (d) impairment of the back, (e) vision impairment, (f) arthritis and rheumatism, (g) diabetes, (h) tuberculosis (TB), (i) heart ailment, (j) hypertension, and (k) cerebrovascular disease. The study revealed that the Filipinos had the highest rate of TB and the lowest rate of arthritis and rheumatism. In all other categories, their rates were intermediate (Burch, 1978).

A 1991 Department of Health study (cited in Weygan-Hildebrand, 1995) indicated that of 213 Filipinos surveyed, 82% considered themselves in excellent or good health. The top ten chronic conditions referred to doctors were hypertension, impairment of back or spine, hayfever without asthma, arthritis/rheumatism, hearing impairment, diabetes, heart condition, chronic and allergic skin condition, asthma without hayfever, and chronic sinusitis. Filipino immigrant health problems such as parasitism and TB were not captured in the statistics. The survey also revealed fewer cases of mental and nervous conditions among Filipinos and Japanese at 6.5 and 8.9 per 1,000 persons, respectively, while among Whites and Hawaiians at 25.3 and 13.2 per 1,000 persons, respectively.

Health Status of Filipino Children

The Hawaii Department of Health survey in 1991 (cited in Weygan-Hildebrand, 1995) revealed youth health problems. According to the study, 18% of the children born in 1991 were from Filipino mothers. Approximately 10% of these births were to babies of low birth weight (less than 2.5 kilograms). Furthermore, 35% of the babies were from mothers who did not go for first trimester prenatal visits. In addition, of the Filipino children born in 1986, only 57% of them were immunized at 24 months, and dental cavities were prevalent among Filipino children (Weygan-Hildebrand, 1995).

In 1995, Nowack, Brozzolara, and Lally conducted a study to measure bone mineral content (BMC) in 86 children, ages 6 to 13 from Hawaiian ($n = 26$), Asian ($n = 42$), Anglo ($n = 11$), and Filipino ($n = 6$) descent. Results revealed an ethnic group's effect on BMC with the Hawaiian children having a significantly higher BMC than their Asian or White counterparts. The findings suggested that ethnic differences can develop early in life. If these differences are carried into adulthood, then this has implications for susceptibility to osteoporosis among the different ethnic groups. Caution must be made when generalizing the results to Filipinos, however, due to the small sample of Filipinos in the study.

Childbearing

In 1954, the Bureau of Public Health Nursing, Department of Health of Hawaii, published a study on 37 rural and 7 urban Filipino families regarding their cultural beliefs and practices during the childbearing period. There were many beliefs and delightful practices presented in this study, for example, the old Filipino custom of tying together the dried umbilical cords of all the family's children to ensure good feelings among the children and a close familial bond. The results indicated that almost all of the present-day folkways about maternity found among Filipinos are not harmful to mother or child. Just two customs might have an untoward effect on the mother: the practice of "extraversion" done by unskilled people and "massage," practiced immediately after delivery for the purpose of retroverting the uterus to prevent future conception. Nurses will find this material useful as a start in orienting them to the Filipino family.

In 1994, Davis, Novotny, Ross, and Wasnich conducted a study comparing the bone mass among women ranging in age from 25 to 34. There were women of Hawaiian ($n = 66$), White ($n = 137$), Japanese ($n = 144$), and Filipino ($n = 74$) descent. The site of bone measurements were at the spine, calcaneus, and proximal and distal radius. The average bone mineral density (BMD) remained stable with age at all four bones sites for the women, indicating the studied age range as representative of peak bone mass. Low bone mass is a major cause of osteoporotic fractures; therefore, differences in bone mass among ethnicities may indicate differences in fracture risk.

The findings revealed that Hawaiian and White women had greater bone measurements than Filipino and Japanese women, largely due to ethnic differences in height and weight as well as calcium intake, exercise, and estrogen and thiazide use. An exception was the greater BMD at the distal radius of Filipino and Japanese women compared to White women. This difference appears to be due to the distribution of the bone mineral across White women's wider bone widths, and might lead to altered risks of distal radius (wrist) fractures. Individual women differed widely in bone mass, regardless of ethnicity, at all four of the bone sites studied (Davis et al., 1994). The researchers concluded that ethnicity is not a good indicator of bone mass for an individual.

Cardiovascular Disease

A study was conducted by Hackenberg, Gerber, and Hackenberg (1978) to investigate whether Filipinos followed the heart disease pattern of people living in the Pacific area, for example, the Japanese, who are exposed for the first time to the full impact of Western urban-industrial society. The data consisted of annual average mortality rates for the five-year period of 1968 through 1972. Of note was that only Filipino male mortality data were utilized. The researchers asked if (a) the mortality rates among Filipinos in Hawaii over time should undergo an increase in coronary heart disease (CHD) and a decrease in cerebrovascular accident (CVA) and (b) rural farm employment within the context of an ethnically homogeneous population was associated with lower rates of CHD (and, perhaps, higher rates of CVA) than urban-industrial employment in a heterogeneous population.

The results confirm that over time CHD rates increased and CVA rates decreased among Filipino male immigrants to Hawaii. An unexpected finding revealed, however, that the Filipino male risk for death due to heart attack appeared to be *lower* than that of the Japanese at the beginning of the interval and *higher* than the comparison group after a mere lapse of 20 years (1950–1970). The findings also confirmed that increasing risks for death from both heart attack and stroke were encountered as Filipinos moved from a rural to an urban environment. The social change was due to the mechanization of the sugar plantations since World War II. The accompanying residential change meant movement from the outer islands to Oahu, primarily to the densely populated parts of the Honolulu metropolitan area.

A study was conducted by Boren (1994) to explore the relationships between value orientations, perceived barriers to and benefits of preventive health behavior, and cardiovascular health risk status in a sample of 61 young Filipino immigrant women with low socioeconomic status. The results revealed that the women valued a traditional family structure, self-development, and planning for change. They perceived more benefits than barriers to preventive health behavior and had a low overall risk for cardiovascular disease. However, 82% of the women had elevated total cholesterol/HDL ratios, 81.9% exercised less than is recommended, 37.7% had central obesity, and 59% reported higher stress levels. Risk factors as such need further investigations.

Unexplained Death

In 1964, Larsen wrote about an incident report in the *Hawaii Medical Journal,* which revealed the death of 120 young strong Filipino men who had gone to bed apparently healthy but who, in the course of the night, were heard to groan, gasp, and die. Larsen compared this incident to similar happenings from other parts of the United States and other countries. For example, 157 young Japanese, mostly males, from 1955 to 1957 also died for no apparent reason. A similar case concerned the death of 19 young Mexican workers who died in their sleep in San Francisco and 140 young American soldiers believed to be in excellent health, who died during World War II. A German study of 2,668 subjects indicated similar results to the World War II study. Larsen concluded that the sudden death for no apparent reason may be attributed to a hypersensitive mechanism of the respiratory center present in certain individuals. This was not unique to the Filipinos. In hypersensitized individuals, minor trauma or sudden emotional stress can cause cessation of breathing and even death. This syndrome was referred to by the French as "death by inhibition."

THE FILIPINO ELDERLY

Assessment and Current Problems

The elderly Filipino in Hawaii mostly came from the barrios of Ilocos Norte or Ilocos Sur. Some had one to two years of education, but most were illiterate. A typical immigrant left home during his or her early twenties, between 1907 and 1931, and was usually single. This Filipino was born without any medical care and received none before coming to the United States. He or she lived in a single-room or shared a substandard shack with other Filipinos in an enclave. Working years were spent as a laborer, and now the Filipino survives on social security supplemented by welfare. Much of the money is sent home to provide education for siblings or children, because the Philippines does not have a system of free education. Often he or she was deprived of a family and individual dreams. In essence, he or she was severed from the social structure which would have provided support, affiliation, and old-age pension. In Hawaii, the Filipino elderly constitute 15% of the population (Hawaii Executive Office on Aging, 1995). Problems of elderly Filipinos reflect their unique history. The average age of the elderly Filipino is 77.

Delayed Marriage. A few Filipino men have saved their meager earnings to return to their homeland to visit and to marry younger women. These May–December unions have created many problems. When the young wives are brought to this country, they experience culture shock and have problems adjusting. They seek jobs to supplement their husband's meager income and leave young children to be cared for by these men in their 70s. In some instances, the men have been confined to nursing homes due to strokes or other infirmities, leaving their wives to cope with child rearing and working in menial jobs. A public health nurse, who has several of these families in her caseload, has reported handicapping and defective conditions among the children, which compounds the already dismal situation. In one family, the husband is 66 and the wife, 34. Their 11-year-old child has flat feet, and the 7-year-old child has congenital esotropia and tests at "dull normal to retarded." In another family, the husband is 71, the wife,

39; their 6-year-old has cleft lip and palate, discrepancy in the length of legs, and malalignment of toes. In yet another family, the husband is 67, the wife, 45. Their 11-year-old has ptosis of the left eyelid with 20/80 vision, and the 8-year-old has inturning of the left foot.

Why do these marriages occur? Each person queried gave varying reasons. Reasons for the elderly male included a need to (a) maintain a genealogical link in having a son, (b) capture the family life one has missed, (c) have someone to care for him when incapacitated, and (d) have normal sex relations. The young wives cited wanting to immigrate to the United States because life in the barrios was harsh and cruel. One young wife, who continually referred to her husband as the father of her child, rather than her husband, said she would like to work and save her money so that she could send for her brother. It seemed that she served as a "sacrificial lamb" for the entire family, making it possible for others in her family to come to the United States.

Health Problems. Dr. Benedict J. Duffy, Jr. contends that elderly Filipinos in the United States are basically healthy or they would not have survived to old age (Spencer & Dorr, 1972). This seems to hold a certain truth for the elderly Filipino men who function well in their daily activities, reported by outreach workers. According to Filipino sources, their attitude toward illness is that unless one is not able to walk or is extremely ill, he or she is not ill.

Screening programs show Filipinos have hypertension, high blood sugar levels, and some gout. The frequency of gout was noted in the literature with accompanying hyperuricemia in Hawaii, Seattle, and Alaska. It is interesting to note that while gout is a relatively rare disease in the Philippines, with an incidence of 0.01%, it has an incidence of 0.68% in Honolulu. Hyperuricemia is not characteristic of the Filipinos in the Philippines. Healey, Skeith, Decker, and Bayam-Sioson, writing in the *American Journal of Human Genetics,* hypothesized that Filipinos are genetically incapable of handling the higher purine loads imposed by a meat-enriched diet characteristic of the United States (Healey et al., 1967). A practicing rheumatologist stated that the Filipinos have high blood uric acid levels, but only about 20% of these have gout; due to a genetic defect, their kidneys do not secrete sufficient uric acid. Many are actually misdiagnosed as having gout because they do not respond to gout treatment. Thus, the Filipinos may have hyperuricemia but the incidence of gout is questionable.

Fisher reported higher incidences of diabetes, TB, syphilis, neurodermatitis, chronic renal disease, high blood pressure, cardiac disease, and elevated hemoglobin levels among Filipino men. He cited race, diet, and stress as contributing to these conditions (Fisher, 1959). Chung Hoon and Hedgcock (1956) reported 24% of 271 new cases of leprosy were among Filipinos born and reared in the Philippines.

The findings of a 1970 Rochester, New York, study indicated that 92% of the general population between the ages of 65 and 69 were able to live alone; this percentage declined sharply after age 75 (Spencer & Dorr, 1972). To extrapolate from this, most of the Filipinos who immigrated between 1907 and 1920 would fall in this latter category and would, therefore, have problems in independent living. A local government intermediate care facility which hospitalizes low socioeconomic level patients registered about 12 elderly Filipino in a census of 200. The caretakers reported having many elderly Filipino patients from time to time. They state that those who were married socialized better; the single men were passive, but enjoyed social groups of single Filipino men with common backgrounds.

The mental health of the Filipino-American elderly is remarkably good, considering difficulties associated with physical disability, poverty, malnutrition, loneliness, few friends, and the poor public attitude toward the elderly. The Rochester study found that 84% of the aged in that community were fully normal mentally (Spencer & Dorr, 1972). However, the California Department of Mental Hygiene reported a disproportionately large number of Filipino men in state mental hospitals. Kalish and Yuen (1971) stated that this may be an indication of the stress experienced by those whose social environment was predictable only in the sense that it was consistently nonsupportive. This may indicate problems of disposition or caretaking. There may be few or no boarding or nursing homes with Filipino caretakers who would care for Filipino men. It is a well-known fact that the elderly are often misplaced in mental institutions because of a lack of other adequate facilities. These early reports need to be updated so that patterns of mental problems in the Filipino-American elders can be traced.

Attitudes Toward Illness and Healthcare.   Although magic and superstition remain an important part of Filipino thinking, the average-age Filipino willingly accepts medical care when offered. He or she may believe the cause of the illness is due to spirits but docilely accepts treatment offered by Western health professionals. However, he or she also will seek the *hilots,* who cure by massage. Herbal medical practices are still carried out, but they are not deterrents to use of Western medical practices.

Sister Grace Dorothy Limm, Director of Ethnic Ministry of the Catholic Diocese of Honolulu, discussed a situation in which a man believed that the spirits, or *mangkukulam,* were after him, causing the sore on his arm. Because he was a fatalist, he failed to seek care. Instead he became highly paranoid, striking out at the refrigerator, thinking it the source of the spirits. He was treated at a mental hospital and later at a community hospital.

The Filipino elderly have been acculturated enough to recognize the efficacy of medical care and will seek it when severely ill. However, they may have problems in the utilization of care for the following reasons: ignorance of such facilities and the benefits of medical insurance; cost of medical care; language problems; and attitude, defining illnesses as only occurring when one is in acute pain, extremely ill, or unable to walk.

FURTHER RESEARCH NEEDS

As previously mentioned, it was difficult to find literature related to the health status of Filipinos. Vance (1995) had previously concurred with past authors, noting that available data are confusing since Filipinos have been lumped together in the literature with Asians, Spanish-speaking people, and "other categories." Most of the literature found on the health status and problems of the Filipinos was outdated, as old as 20 years. Furthermore, there is a lack of research on the various developmental stages (e.g., childhood, adolescence). Not much research has been done on Filipino women either. For example, the following questions could be investigated:

Why is low birth weight prevalent among Filipino babies?

What causes the high incidence of dental cavities among Filipino children?

What are the healthcare needs of Filipino adolescents?

What are the health problems of Filipino adolescents?

What are the healthcare needs of Filipino women?

Why do Filipino mothers not attend first trimester prenatal visits?

Regarding elderly Filipinos, the following areas could be further researched:

What is the extent of their health problems?

What are their patterns of healthcare utilization?

What are their problems in utilization of healthcare?

How many are able to maintain independent living and until what age?

What is their standard of living?

What are concurrent problems with those men who were reunited with families after a 20-year absence?

What are the disposition problems when independent living is no longer possible?

What are their coping mechanisms in light of meager support systems?

What are their nutritional differences and their effect on hyperuricemia?

What are cross-cultural findings from longevity studies of Filipino men who immigrated to the United States versus those who did not?

What are the stress factors and disease conditions?

From the authors' own experiences, the World War II Filipino veterans, now in their 70s and 80s, came to Hawaii with much hope of bringing their families to the United States. Because of their advanced age, they cannot work and are often hospitalized for various chronic problems. Since they have no medical insurance, this places a burden on the family that sponsored them as well as on the U.S. health system that is already in flux. Therefore, research questions related to coping, access to healthcare, and caregivers of this new group of immigrants need further investigation.

REFERENCES

Boren, D. M. (1994). *Value orientations, barriers and benefits, and cardiovascular disease risk in young Filipino women.* (Thesis). University of Hawaii.

Burch, T. A. (1978). *Ethnicity and health in Hawaii, 1975.* Research and Statistics Office, Hawaii State Department.

Bureau of Public Health Nursing. (1954). *Cultural beliefs and practices of the childbearing period and their implications for nursing practice: Among Chinese, Filipino, Hawaiian, and Japanese families living in Hawaii.* Hawaii.

Chung Hoon, E. K. M., & Hedgcock, G. (1956). Racial aspects of leprosy and recent therapeutic advantages. *Hawaii Medical Journal, 16*(2), 125-130.

Davis, J. W., Novotny, R., Ross, P. D., & Wasnich, R. D. (1994). The peak bone mass of Hawaiian, Filipino, Japanese, and White women living in Hawaii. *Calcified Tissue International, 55*(4), 249-252.

Executive Office on Aging. (1995). *Three year plan.* Honolulu, HI: Author.

Fisher, H. W. (1959). The diseases of the Filipino men. *Hawaii Medical Journal, 18*(3), 252-254.

Hackenberg, R. A., Gerber, L., & Hackenberg, B. H. (1978). *Cardiovascular disease mortality among Filipinos in Hawaii: Rates, trends, and associated factors.* Research and Statistics Office, Hawaii State Department of Health.

Healey, L. A., Skeith, M. D., Decker, J. L., & Bayam-Sioson, P. S. (1967). Hyperuricemia in Filipinos: Interaction of heredity and environment. *American Journal of Human Genetics, 19*(2), 81–85.

Jones, G. B. (1974). *People and cultures in Hawaii.* Honolulu: University of Hawaii School of Medicine.

Kalish, R., & Yuen, S. (1971, Spring). Americans of the East-American ancestry: Aging and the aged. *The Gerontologist, Part II,* 36–47.

Kroeber, A. L. (1928). Peoples of the Philippines (2nd ed.). New York: Anthropological Handbook Fund.

Larsen, N. P. (1964). Sudden death of Filipino men in Hawaii. *Journal of the National Medical Association, 56*(1), 52–54.

Lasker, B. (1940). Filipinos in California. *Amerasia, 3,* 575–579.

Ledesma, B. (1976, February). The Filipinos: The people who came and stayed. *Foundation of History and Humanities Cultural Camp* handout at camp held at Kualoa Beach Park.

Nowack, M. K., Brozzolara, S., & Lally, D. A. (1995). Bone mineral content in Hawaiian, Asian, and Filipino children. *Hawaii Medical Journal, 54*(1), 388–389, 393.

San Buanaventura, S. (1995). *Filipino immigration to the U.S.* The Asian American Encyclopedia. New York: Marshall Cavendish.

Spencer, M. G., & Dorr, C. J. (1972). *Understanding aging: A multi-disciplinary approach.* New York: Appleton-Century-Crofts.

U.S. Department of Commerce, Bureau of Census. (1993a). *Population profile of the United States* (Publication No. 23-185). Washington, DC: U.S. Government Printing Office.

U.S. Department of Commerce, Bureau of Census. (1993b, September). *We the Americana . . . Asians.* Washington, DC: U.S. Government Printing Office.

Vance, A. R. (1995). Filipino Americans. In J. N. Giger & R. E. Davidhizar (Eds.), *Transcultural nursing, assessment and intervention* (2nd ed., pp. 416–438). St. Louis: Mosby.

Weygan-Hildebrand, C. (1995). *A snapshot about Filipinos in Hawaii.* Hawaii Community Foundation Diversity Project. Partially funded by a grant from the Ford Foundation. Hawaii.

Zabilka, G. (1970). *Customs and cultures of the Philippines.* Rutland, VT: Charles E. Tuttle.

Zaide, G. F. (1937). *Early Philippine history and culture.* Oriental Printing.

Zamora, M. D. (1967). *Studies in Philippine Anthropology.* Quezon City, Philippines: Alema-Phoenix.

CHAPTER SEVEN

The Invisible Disease: HIV/AIDS in Asian Americans

Jillian Inouye, PhD, RN

HIV/AIDS is the invisible disease in Asian Americans. Because of low incidence reports; a lack of data and documentation; a large number of subgroups; and sociocultural, linguistic, and environmental barriers, HIV/AIDS has been largely ignored in a mainstream American healthcare system. During the early years of the AIDS epidemic, the number of reported cases among Asian Americans was small compared to other racial groups. Asians were often presumed to be at a lesser risk than other groups, and this led to complacency because people believed that acquired immune deficiency syndrome (AIDS) was not a problem within their Asian communities. Although Asian Americans are small in number, it is estimated that along with the Pacific Island population, it is the fastest growing group in the United States. By the year 2050, the projection is for Asian Americans to increase by 356%, making them 11% (41 million) of the U.S. population (Lin-Fu, 1993). This large increase has implications as the numbers affected by this disease continue to grow (Woo, Rutherford, Payne, Barnhart, & Lemp, 1988).

Another problem in surveying the complexity of HIV/AIDS in Asian Americans is the inadequate documentation of data. Unfortunately, data on HIV/AIDS are not collected separately for the different Asian ethnic groups in the United States. Because they are combined in most statistical and epidemiological reports and because of the diverse Asian racial and ethnic subgroups, it is difficult to know exactly the scope of the problem in the various ethnic groups.

Furthermore, Asian Americans are often neglected by researchers because of a conspiracy of silence and cultural beliefs. Denial, shame, and privacy concerns associated with AIDS prevent those with the disease from revealing their status to friends and family. Misconceptions that Asians are not at risk for HIV and that homosexuality is not common also inhibit discussion and information sharing. Moreover, language difficulties impede effective communication. To shed more light on this topic and dispel the myth of the model minority regarding health needs, this chapter will outline the problems of HIV/AIDS in the Asian American community, review the literature, and recommend possible actions.

METHODOLOGY

A review of the literature was completed for the years 1987 through 1997 utilizing the following databases: MEDLINE, AIDSLINE, CINHL, Uncover, and Psychological Abstracts. Search keywords included (a) *HIV or AIDS* and *Asian and Americans*, (b) *HIV or AIDS* and *Asian and American or Japanese or Chinese or Korean or Filipino or Thai or Hmong,* and (c) *Asian and Health.* More than 1,471 documents were retrieved. Most articles were related to health education programs for Asian Americans or the results of knowledge, attitudes, beliefs, and behaviors (KABB) studies. Many were abstracts from the International Conferences on AIDS. Only 83 addressed Asian Americans and of those only 42 concerned Asian Americans with HIV/AIDS.

SCOPE OF THE PROBLEM

While Asians and Pacific Islanders are two distinct groups, the U.S. Census Bureau and other agencies combine the two in health statistics and census counts. There are more than 28 Asian subgroups and 20 Pacific Islander subgroups (U.S. Bureau of the Census, 1992). Within the Asian group, Chinese and Filipinos are the two largest subgroups followed by Japanese, Asian Indians, and Koreans. Combined with the Pacific Islanders, this group is projected to reach 41 million, or 10.7% of the population (U.S. Bureau of the Census, 1992). Because of this combination, it is often difficult to determine ethnic-specific health problems and exact numbers.

According to the Centers for Disease Control (CDC, 1994), there was a cumulative total of 767 reported AIDS cases in Asian-Pacific Americans (API) in the United States. While seemingly the lowest rate compared to other ethnic groups, the annual rate of increase parallels that of others. According to the National AIDS Network (1989), the incidence of AIDS among API was doubling about every 10 months between 1992 and 1993. Newly reported cases of AIDS among API increased 129%, compared to 117% among Whites. Homosexual or bisexual contacts accounted for 72% of all Asian AIDS cases (CDC, 1994). A study by California's Office of AIDS (Jew, 1991) found different incidence rates among ethnic groups. This ranged from a high of 66.5 cases per 100,000 for Thais to a low of 2.7 cases per 100,000 for people of Korean origin. The second to lowest rate was the Vietnamese at 6.4 cases per 100,000.

In San Diego there was a 171% increase in AIDS cases among API between 1993 and 1994 (County of San Diego, 1994). The city now has the second highest HIV seroprevalence rate in the state of California (Loue, Lloyd, & Loh, 1996).

Woo and associates' (1988) survey of AIDS in Asian and Pacific Islander populations in San Francisco found the incidence of AIDS in this group significantly lower than Whites (1,108 per 100,000) at 58.5 cases per 100,000. However, AIDS cases among API in San Francisco have increased 177% since 1985, compared with 54% in other racial and ethnic groups. This has been an alarming and rapid increase. Filipinos accounted for 42%; Chinese, 21%; Japanese, 21%; Polynesian, 6%; and Southeast Asian, 5% of the API. Eighty-three percent were homosexual or bisexual men without histories of intravenous (IV) drug use, 7% were transfusion recipients, and 4% were heterosexual drug users. A significantly greater proportion of cases involved transfusion recipients in the API group versus the non-API group. Increasing incidence was found in gay and bisexual men and suggests HIV entered the API homosexual and bisexual communities later than the non-API and may thus show increased numbers at a later date. Woo and associates further report that the incidence of AIDS was 141 cases per 100,000 Japanese, 92 per 100,000 Filipinos, 72 per 100,000 southeast Asians, and 21 per 100,000 Chinese. Forty-seven percent involved Filipinos while they represent only 26% of the State's Asian American population. However, Japanese Americans suffer a higher incidence of AIDS in contrast to Filipinos, Vietnamese, and Chinese when adjusted for size of their community (Ja & Ngin, 1987). The Filipino and Japanese Americans who settled in urban areas in large numbers have shown high incidences of HIV infection and AIDS (Aoki, Ngin, Mo, & Ja, 1989).

In a prevalence study of HIV infection in a sample of immigrants, Studemeister and Kent (1993) found the HIV infection rate of people applying for U.S. permanent residence comparable to, if not less than, that of the general American population, and lower than the seroprevalence rates of persons in high-risk groups such as gay men and IV drug injectors. This rate of seroprevalence varied depending on the region of origin, with immigrants from the Caribbean having the highest (2.44%) and those from Asian communities the lowest (0.05%). Studemeister and Kent state the findings do not necessarily reflect HIV seroprevalence rates of the regions since immigrants may have become infected while residing in the United States.

Metler, Hu, Fleming, and Ward (1994) found that 1,358 of API born outside of the United States accounted for 59% of all cases among API in San Francisco, Los Angeles, and New York City. Those with AIDS born outside of the United States predominantly originated from the Philippines (29%), Japan (7%), China (6%), Vietnam (6%), India (5%), and Thailand (5%).

In Hawaii, Asians and Pacific Islanders account for 62% of Hawaii's population and 26% of cumulative AIDS cases (State of Hawaii, 1997). The case rates per 100,000 populations for Hawaii's Chinese, Filipino, and Japanese populations are 9.0, 7.2, and 4.5, respectively. In the five years between 1986 and 1990, 28% of cumulative AIDS patients were non-Whites, and between 1991 and 1995 this figure increased to 39% (AIDS Community Care Team & The Governor's Committee on HIV/AIDS, 1996). The epidemic in Hawaii, mirroring the U.S. mainland, is spreading among the ethnic populations in the state and others with high concentrations of Asian groups.

TRANSMISSION PATTERNS

Gock (1994) suggests that the prevalent mode of transmission of HIV for APIs is through male-male sexual contacts versus IV drug use. This is similar to that of Whites as opposed to other ethnic minority groups. Confirming his suggestion, new AIDS cases among homosexual API increased 55% between 1989 and 1994 compared with 14% for White gay men (CDC, 1995). The infection rate was higher among API gay men (26.9%) comported to White gay men (15.5%) (Osmond, Page, Wiley, et al., 1994). In addition, the CDC acknowledged that the number of reported cases may actually represent an underestimation of prevalence due to cultural and other factors which prevent an accurate count of cases in this community. Gock (1994) surmises that the cultural factors related to low reporting of infection are related to shame, loss of face at contracting a socially stigmatized disease, delay of reporting by private practice physicians, and misdiagnosis by folk practitioners visited or utilized by immigrants.

Sidhu, Weinstock, and Gwinn (1996) recently surveyed 3,196 APIs tested for HIV/AIDS in San Francisco, Los Angeles, Houston, and Boston and found a surprisingly high proportion (25%) of the males had sex with other men although seroprevalence decreased in this group from 31% between 1990 and 1992 to 17% between 1993 and 1994. Nevertheless, they felt the high rates were of particular concern with necessary education and prevention programs needed.

BARRIERS TO CARE

The Workgroup on Barriers to HIV Care for Asians and Pacific Islanders (1994) met May 9 through May 10 and identified and categorized common barriers to care according to the following categories: cultural, structural, and "other" barriers. Cultural barriers included diversity, negotiating the healthcare system, service providers, and the public belief of AIDS as being a gay disease. Structural barriers included lack of technical assistance, data collection problems and funding levels, limitations of aggregating data, limited infrastructure of Asian and Pacific Islander agencies, network of API service providers, and lack of policy representations. "Other" barriers included lack of services for women, inadequate youth services, inefficient systems within agencies, clinical trials, lack of access to alternative treatment, insensitivity among providers, and barriers within AIDS education and training centers. These barriers are discussed as they relate to Asian Americans.

Cultural Barriers

Cultural barriers can be examined using the dimension of individualism-collectivism (Hofstede, 1984). Western cultures have been conceptualized as individualistic cultures where individual goals and concerns are emphasized. Collectivism, which is common with Asian Pacific Islanders, emphasizes group goals and concerns. This collectivistic orientation draws a distinction between in-groups and out-groups. The past stigmatization of AIDS as a homosexual disease preys on the concept of individualism-collectivism in the Asian community. Because of the low incidence of and reporting of homosexuality, AIDS is often perceived as an out-group disease, resulting in people's lack of concern regarding their risk status.

There are strong taboos against open discussions or exhibition of sexuality and heavy stigmatization of homosexuality (Aoki, Ngin, Mo, & Ja, 1989). The Asian expectation is of the male, especially the firstborn, to marry and perpetuate the family name. Homosexuality brings family dishonor and possible ostracism by the family and community (Choi, Salazar, Lew, & Coates, 1995). This leads to a further lack of direct communication and self-disclosure about sexual behavior. The reduction of interpersonal communication affects exchange of information about AIDS in the Asian communities, leads to increased isolation, and reduces the effectiveness of educational and health promotion programs.

Research focusing on these barriers include work by Brown (1992) who conducted a survey with Asian-Pacific Islander and White students. He found that while there was no gender difference regarding respondents' knowledge of AIDS, there were significant differences between Whites and Asian-Pacific Islanders. The API expressed less personal concern and engaged in less interpersonal communication about AIDS. This lack of concern and interpersonal communication lulls the group into a lack of personal concern about contracting AIDS and reduces effectiveness of educational messages about sexual relationships and AIDS.

Included in this conspiracy of silence are healthcare workers. Gellert and colleagues (1994) report anecdotal information indicating that some Asian physicians treat STDs without laboratory diagnoses to ensure client confidentiality without breaching disease reporting laws. This practice, they state, can reduce motivation for HIV testing by those with confirmed STDs.

Structural Barriers

Asian Americans consist of approximately 28 subgroups with 32 linguistic groups. Lack of knowledge about the differences in subgroups and inconsistencies in coding for race and ethnicity in health statistics contribute to myths regarding the health of the Asian population. It is extremely difficult to determine exact numbers and specific health problems because of increasing intermarriage and ethnicity coding according to a hierarchy of categories. For example, a child with Asian and African American parents would be classified as African American. This adds to the difficulty of developing health policy and programs for Asian Americans.

Other Barriers

Asian gay women and men have problems related to their gender and sexual status. Their reliance on care is primarily on the formal systems of healthcare. Because of the collectivism and lack of communication about their problems, they lack the informal community networks of support—tangible and emotional—that gay White men have developed. Especially for Asian women, HIV carries the added burden of isolation in a social system different from that of men. As one Asian woman stated, "I feel like I'm the only Japanese woman with HIV in Hawaii." Kitano (1988) reports that Asians in general "do not want their families and community to know that they have AIDS because it means that their sexual preference may become known. . . . They don't want to risk being rejected at a time when they are in need nor do they want to 'shame' their families" (p. 4). This fear and shame apply to men and women alike.

Clinical trials in the United States have consisted mainly of middle-class, married White males. An extensive review by Swanson and Ward (1995) on recruiting minorities into all types of clinical trials identified four barriers to recruitment and participation. These included sociocultural, economic, individual, and research. Sociocultural barriers include racial and ethnic discrimination as well as differences in health beliefs and health behaviors. Economic barriers included the lack of access to healthcare in general. This covered poor quality of services and poverty, which limited access. Denial and underestimation of personal vulnerability were listed as individual barriers to participation in research. Research barriers included those related to the study design, researcher bias, and the small percentage of minority healthcare professionals. Under study design are restrictive exclusion criteria, differences in drug response, and complexity of forms and procedures. Research biases included failure to accommodate cultural and economic diversity, fear of lack of statistical power loss, belief that certain populations are not at risk for illnesses, and the claim that minorities are "hard to research." Lack of a large enough number of minority healthcare professionals, which minorities tend to utilize because of general distrust of academic medicine, is another difficulty encountered in clinical trials. These barriers to clinical trials seem inclusive for treatment and education programs as well.

RESEARCH FINDINGS

Most of the research on HIV/AIDS and Asian Americans has utilized KABB surveys of non-infected or high-risk individuals. Very few have involved actual infected individuals. Because of the overlap of knowledge, attitudes, and beliefs, they are discussed together and risk behaviors are discussed separately.

Knowledge–Attitudes–Beliefs

One of the earliest studies was done by DiClemente, Zorn, and Temoshok (1987). They found ethnic differences in knowledge about AIDS, with Asians having lower overall knowledge than Hispanics, Blacks, and Whites. A similar telephone survey in the Chicago area by Albrecht and colleagues (1989) found that being of Hispanic or Asian origin meant one was less likely to have heard about AIDS. Another telephone survey in Massachusetts (Strunin, 1991) probing beliefs, attitudes, and behaviors of adolescents about AIDS found that Asians knew significantly less than other groups about sexual and drug use transmission of the virus. Yet they were significantly more worried about getting AIDS and thought that they would get it.

Another telephone survey of 1,540 adults, of which 47 (3%) were Asians (Prohaska, Albrecht, Levy, Sugrue, & Kim, 1990), found Asian Americans and persons with no particular religious affiliation report greater perceptions of risk. Despite the low recorded infection rate, they felt that this response reflected the view that Asians perceive the AIDS virus as contagious as smallpox, tuberculosis (TB), and malaria (Aoki et al., 1989).

Hingson et al. (1991) administered a questionnaire about knowledge regarding HIV transmission, beliefs, and risky health practices to 3,049 Boston middle and high school students. They found that immigrant students were more likely to worry about getting AIDS. They were less likely to talk to their parents about AIDS and to know ways of avoiding transmission, where to obtain information, and where to be tested for HIV. They also were more likely to have misconceptions about transmission. They believed that no one their age used condoms if sexually active and that most people their ages were injecting drugs. These immigrant students were less likely to report having sexual intercourse, but of those who were active, a higher percentage reported having sex with an IV drug user. A large proportion (62%) of sexually active adolescents did not consistently use condoms.

Goh (1993) surveyed 274 students attending City University of New York. The sample included 50 Asians born in the United States with family histories of at least two generations and recent immigrant Asians, as well as other ethnic groups. He found a greater proportion of Whites, Blacks, and Hispanics rating themselves as knowledgeable or very knowledgeable about HIV/AIDS as compared to the recent immigrant Asians who were the least knowledgeable. Television, lectures and workshops on AIDS, everyday conversations, and contact with people with AIDS were attended to significantly less by the Asian group.

Gellert et al. (1995) more recently surveyed 532 California Vietnamese on their knowledge and attitudes about HIV/AIDS and self-reported sexual and other high-risk practices. While knowledge about modes of transmission was generally accurate, a substantial minority believed that HIV could be transmitted through casual contact and from needles in hospitals. Twenty-nine percent did not believe they would be infected and almost one-half felt they did not have enough information about AIDS to protect themselves. While no same-sex behavior was reported, 6% of the men had visited a female prostitute, and a large percent of sexually active unmarried respondents reported they never use (17%–40%) or only sometimes use (10%–32%) condoms.

Loue et al. (1996) conducted a focus group with a convenience sample of 282 API respondents. They matched interviewers by gender and either language or ethnicity to increase the comfort level of the respondents. In addition, a questionnaire was given to determine attitudes, knowledge, and risk behaviors. Results of the focus group indicate that many APIs prefer obtaining their healthcare from API healthcare workers but that these providers rarely discussed risk behaviors for HIV and other sexually transmitted diseases. They also rarely provided them with information about how to prevent HIV and where to obtain testing. The questionnaire further revealed that the majority of respondents could not identify a medically accepted cause of HIV transmission and only 24% had been tested for HIV—despite the presence of risk factors for HIV transmission, such as unprotected visits to prostitutes (25.2%) and sexual relations with multiple partners (23.7%). Seventeen percent believed that the diagnosis of HIV must be made by physicians and could not be made on the basis of blood tests. More respondents (54.3%) indicated they might accept a condom from their physician or other healthcare provider but not from a street distribution program and that seeing a doctor was a preferred mode for initial treatment of any illness.

Risk Behaviors

Risk factors associated with transmission and exposure to HIV generally include sexual behaviors and drug use. High-risk sexual activities include multiple partners; unprotected anal, vaginal, and oral sex; bondage and discipline; and anal play. High-risk drug use includes sharing needles, using contaminated needles, and drinking alcohol. Cultural pressures such as a tendency for sexual conservatism, less discussion about sex, reserved display of strong emotions, reluctance to disrupt the social order, and maintenance of family unity previously helped to reduce the occurrence of risk behaviors among Asian Americans (Hirayama & Hirayama, 1986). Indeed, some researchers (Cochran, Mays, & Leung, 1991) have found a lower rate of sexual activity in Asian Americans (47%) compared to Whites (72%), Blacks (84%), and Hispanics (59%). Yet like other young adults, Asians also practice risky behaviors, such as failing to use condoms and engaging in sexual behaviors that will transmit HIV.

While low rates had been previously reported for API between 1989 and 1990, the greatest proportional increase in AIDS cases has now been noted among API (Toleran, 1991). Asian American college students reported lower rates of sexual activity; however, once active their risk-taking behavior patterns are similar to those of young adults in other ethnic groups (Cochran et al., 1991). To compare risk behaviors among Whites, Chinese, and Filipino American adolescents in San Francisco, Horan and DiClemente (1993) used the CDC surveillance study. They found only 13% of the Chinese sample to be sexually active while 32% of the Filipino sample and 37% of the White sample were active. There were no differences regarding drug use behaviors. Chinese students indicated significantly less ability to communicate with others about HIV disease and prevention and along with the Filipino students, had fewer misconceptions about HIV knowledge but less knowledge about HIV prevention than White students. Because of differences in sexual activity within the Asian ethnic groups, certain groups may be at greater risk than others due to poor communication and less HIV prevention information.

Carrier, Nguyen, and Su's (1992) field research data on Vietnamese American sexual behaviors indicate that the potential exists for the spread of HIV into the heterosexual Vietnamese population through sexual activity of Vietnamese men with non-Vietnamese female prostitutes in California and Mexico and with Thai and Vietnamese prostitutes in Thailand and Vietnam. There is greater risk related to males having sexual encounters with other men because of the high level of homophobia, community members' reluctance to be tested for HIV, and the underreporting of cases.

Yep's (1992-1993) extensive review of the literature based on the risk reduction model in the API community found the following:

1. Most of the APIs had lower HIV knowledge scores than their ethnic peers, particularly in the area of casual transmission.
2. Regarding susceptibility to HIV infection, studies were inconclusive with some reporting that APIs are more concerned about HIV infection than other ethnic groups while others report the contrary.
3. There were several cultural norms operating relating to risk, such as sexual conservatism, strong negative attitudes toward homosexuality, bisexuality, drug use, and avoidance of discussion of topics such as sexual behavior, homosexuality, illness and death.
4. Social support is provided by the family with many finding it difficult to rely on community services or unrelated friends for caretaking activities.
5. Asian men viewed safe sexual practices as extremely effective for prevention.
6. APIs consistently underutilize health related services and were less willing to discuss HIV/AIDS with a new sexual partner.

A large ($n = 874$) study in California focusing on Vietnamese indicated that HIV infection exists and men who have sex with men appear to be at risk for HIV infection similar to others practicing high-risk behaviors (Gellert, Moore, Maxwell, Mai, & Higgins, 1994). A convenience sample of 241 self-identified gay API men in San Francisco (Choi, Coates, Catania, Lew, & Chow, 1995) revealed a high level of AIDS knowledge but only 17% believed that they were at risk for HIV infection. Most men reported multiple sexual partners (95%) and engaging in unprotected sex (27%), as compared to previous reports of 18% by Ekstrand and Coates (1990). These data highlight the high risk for HIV in gay API with the urgent need for multilevel interventions.

Loue, Lloyd, and Phoombour (1994) reported a survey of 165 APIs' knowledge, beliefs, and practices. They found that treatment by a physician was sought primarily in cases of extreme pain (11.5%) or illness of long duration (32.7%), reinforcing the notion that Asians are stoic and seek healthcare only when their illness is very serious. The survey also revealed a relatively low rate of HIV testing (23.6%) despite frequent reports of unprotected sex with multiple partners (72.7%), again reinforcing previous findings of inconsistent beliefs and postponement of testing and treatment in this group.

In summary, it appears that Asian Americans, unlike their self-identified gay men and lesbian cohorts, are less knowledgeable about HIV disease and transmission than other ethnic groups and maintain many of their cultural beliefs, behaviors, and communication patterns. This is particularly troublesome because the cultural stigma and homophobia make it difficult to target this group for educational programs.

Education/Health Promotion Approaches

Studies on different educational or health promotion approaches include mainly non-infected Asian or Asian American students. The studies summarized in the following section generally dealt with KABB in students or healthcare workers.

An educational program consisting of a slide-tape presentation, an AIDS educational brochure, and a community resource brochure were developed to determine the effects on knowledge, attitudes, and practices for Vietnamese women. Flaskerud and Nyamathi (1988) utilized a control and an experimental group to study this educational intervention. While no differences were found between the control and experimental groups in response to individual items on the questionnaire, significant differences occurred in pretest and posttest scores for the experimental group on most items. There were major changes related to the donation of blood; attitudes toward gay and bisexual men; the subject of children with AIDS; and intended practices including use of condoms, injected drugs, and multiple sexual partners. These results revealed that knowledge of AIDS was generally high and suggest that information can change attitudes and intended changes in practice, at least in the short term.

Horan and DiClemente (1993) found Chinese and Filipino-American students more receptive to general information about modes of transmission than they are to prevention because of sexual and drug use information. Therefore, more time should be spent in overcoming cultural communication barriers regarding discussion of these topics. Horan and DiClemente suggest dividing students by gender when providing specific information on sexual behaviors and using more indirect communication patterns.

Yep (1993a) reported results of a community-based HIV/AIDS education and prevention program for Asians and Pacific Islanders funded by the County of Los Angeles' AIDS Program Office. The three objectives of the program were as follows:

1. Adoption of at least one safer sexual behavior by 70% of the participants.
2. Demonstration of correct use of condoms by 70% of the participants.
3. Demonstration of superior competence (80% accuracy) on an HIV knowledge posttest.

All the objectives were accomplished. The program was a success and recommended methods for health educators to develop education and prevention outreach programs for API communities were proposed.

Loue et al. (1996) developed an educational intervention program for HIV prevention for API through healthcare workers. They formulated their program based on gathered data indicating that APIs had a low level of knowledge relating to risk factors for HIV transmission, risk behaviors for HIV transmission exist within their community, and healthcare providers and physicians specifically are perceived as authoritative figures to be trusted. The program comprised four components:

1. A symposium for healthcare workers.
2. A culturally sensitive and appropriate HIV related video for the healthcare workers and their patients.
3. Ongoing training for the healthcare providers.
4. Ongoing liaison and consultative services for the healthcare providers.

While they received positive qualitative evaluation of the program, no program effectiveness measures have been collected so far.

The only study that looked at differential treatment effects of pharmacy was done by Gibaldi (1993). He found evidence that suggested minority patients may respond differently than Whites to Zidovudine. Though inconclusive, this raises serious concerns regarding the paucity of information about therapeutic benefits and safety of drugs to non-Whites.

HIV-Infected Asian Americans

A few studies involving HIV-infected individuals that did not focus on knowledge, attitudes, beliefs, and behaviors are summarized in this section. These studies have been primarily descriptive in nature.

A focus group utilizing staff and clients was conducted by the Asian and Pacific Islander Coalition for HIV/AIDS, Inc. (APICHA) (Eckholdt,

Chin, Manzon, & Kim, 1994). It recommended that although language was a barrier to service provision, what was needed was access to multiple organizations, and multisite organizations that were physically and socially outside the community.

A study (Yoshioka, Chin, & Manzon, 1996) of 20 interviews with APIs with HIV/AIDS in New York City revealed that participants were concerned with the perceived quality of practical support (i.e., financial assistance). They also considered whether disclosure of their status would cause pain to family and its degree of AIDS phobia. In addition, participants considered language accessibility and cultural competence of staff for institutional support essential.

A counseling study (Choi et al., 1996) conducted on the efficacy of brief group counseling with API gay men found that counseling based on the Health Belief Model was able to reduce risk behaviors in this group. The researchers found a reduction in the number of sexual partners and instances of unprotected anal intercourse after the treatment.

Looking at prevalence of AIDS-defining conditions by race and ethnicity, Hu et al. (1995) found extrapulmonary tuberculosis higher in APIs and other minority groups than among Whites. Metler et al. (1994) found APIs 1.2 times more likely than other racial/ethnic groups combined to have pneumocystic carinii pneumonia (PCP) and 1.7 times more likely to have cytomegalovirus (CMV) retinitis, but only 0.6 times as likely to have HIV encephalopathy. The incidence of pulmonary TB was 2.5 times higher and extrapulmonary TB 3.1 times higher in APIs than that of Whites with AIDS.

RECOMMENDATIONS

Reports on incidence, transmission modes, knowledge, attitudes, beliefs, and behaviors point to the clear risk of Asian American groups for HIV. The review of the literature agrees that strategies employed for prevention, education, and treatment should be linguistically, culturally, and gender appropriate as well as take into consideration a person's sexual orientation. Many Asians are immigrant or foreign born with English as their second language. This increases difficulty in the provision of educational programs. Cultural traditions such as filial respect, maintenance of social order, and cohesiveness still exist in Asian Americans of several generations (Moore & Erikson, 1985). These traditions have a strong impact on health behaviors. For example, behaviors and attitudes from their culture are still present, such as a dislike for blood sampling and other invasive procedures (e.g., pelvic examinations and pap smears in unmarried women) and hospitalization (Lin-Fu, 1993). Attitudes such as shame, denial, and homophobia prevent gay men from disclosing their risk status and heterosexuals from seeking information. Other models of disease and treatment are present with this group, such as the notions of harmony and hot and cold, and the theory of yin and yang. These need to be considered when planning education and treatment programs. Human suffering is still seen as a part of life by some Asian Americans, and stoicism and restraint of public display of emotions are valued. This often leads to postponement of healthcare until symptoms are more severe than the average healthcare seeker as was found in the survey by Loue et al. (1994).

When recommending education, health promotion, and research programs, is it no wonder professionals have difficulty meeting all these criteria for culturally competent care? What follows are recommendations based on a review of information known about Asian Americans. They are divided into two sections: culturally competent education and health promotion and research needs.

Culturally Competent Education and Health Promotion

Communication Issues. Lack of knowledge is surprising to most literate English speakers considering all the money and media spent in our nation's campaign against HIV/AIDS. However, what is often overlooked is the diversity of languages, beliefs, and customs. These campaigns which have a largely North American cultural orientation, and are predominantly in English, are ineffectively reaching the conscience of the API population due to cultural variabilities (Brown, 1992). One must also consider the fact that not all Asians are literate. Many of the immigrants in this country are not only monolingual, but also illiterate in their own native language. Special efforts must be made to reach these new Americans, for analysis of reported AIDS cases among APIs in Los Angeles revealed that more than two-thirds of them were first-generation, foreign-born Asian-Pacific Americans and that it is primarily non-English speaking API immigrants who tend to have the lowest level of accurate AIDS related information (Gock, 1994). Multilingual HIV/AIDS information and healthcare providers are essential steps toward reaching a great segment of the API community, not only ensuring the correct information is disseminated, but also making the non-English speaker feel at ease in our Western healthcare system.

How we present HIV/AIDS information to the Asian population also plays a critical role in its accommodation into the community. This information must not only be linguistically sensitive but also culturally sensitive. In a culture with traditional values based on family and group orientation, self-identification lies heavily within one's own community. Previously discussed studies showed that Asian American students believed AIDS to be a very serious disease but did not personally feel they were susceptible to it, perceiving AIDS and HIV related conditions to be a non-Asian epidemic. In order to increase their self-perceived threat of HIV and thereby decrease the number of risk behaviors by APIs, we must appeal to their sense of community. A simple means may be the addition of Asian models to posters or brochures containing AIDS related information. However, to effectively get the message about AIDS across to APIs, a link must be made between HIV services and education and social institutions within the API community. Help should be solicited from community gatekeepers, particularly the respected health-care professionals and others (i.e., religious leaders, teachers, parents, service providers, and HIV-positive API) as spokespersons and models for HIV prevention (Yep, 1993a). Although there are few HIV-positive APIs who might be willing to come forward publicly with their illness, having them speak out to their own community might, in fact, be the most effective way of showing AIDS to be a very real disease.

Although great strides have been taken to create linguistically and culturally appropriate HIV/AIDS education and prevention materials, health educators and outreach groups have had extreme difficulty in reaching Asian and Pacific Islanders through traditional modes of information dissemination. In Yep's (1993b) summary of the first Asian/Pacific Island Men's HIV Conference in Los Angeles, he felt HIV advertisements in bars were "conventional" channels of information with the gay and lesbian communities—a method which fails to reach homosexual API because most do not openly participate within that community. A survey conducted at a Southern California forum on "Cultural Factors in HIV/AIDS Education and Prevention for Asian and Pacific Islanders: A Multidisciplinary Exploration" found that beauty parlors, bowling alleys, malls, churches and temples, schools, and gambling facilities were "ideal places to investigate the needs of the API community" (Yep 1994, p. 184). Other suggestions might be to target ethnic eateries. Yep provided examples of culturally appropriate strategies that have been quite successful among certain API groups— mainly the use of fortune cookies and the Chinese red envelopes as discreet, nonthreatening, non-Western approaches to AIDS education and the distribution of condoms, dental dams, lubricants, and safer sex information. Of course, what works within the Chinese community may not be effective within another API ethnic group. Each group must make the effort to meet with its own cultural and community figures to discuss strategies and methods for AIDS education and the distribution of information. Privacy and low risk of embarrassment are crucial values to consider with any API group. One other idea to keep in mind when working with Asian and Pacific Islanders is that they would be more likely to attend an information session or accept information on *health* and *lifestyles* rather than *AIDS, HIV, disease,* or *illness.* The words we use as educators must not make them uncomfortable and unreceptive to the importance of our message.

By far, one of the biggest contributing factors to the lack of AIDS knowledge among Asians is probably the cultural reluctance of speaking about sex and AIDS related behaviors. As Gock (1994, p. 260) put it, "Within cultures that are historically reticent to talk about sex and sexuality (not to mention same-gender sexual behaviors and diversity in sexual orientations), to acknowledge the presence of substance abuse among its community members, and to discuss death and dying openly, any attempt to mention any of these three areas, let alone all of them together, is no small feat." This is supported by Loue et al. (1996), who found healthcare providers of API background rarely discussed risk behaviors and other STD concerns with their patients. Clearly, opening the lines of communication between API healthcare providers and patients is of utmost importance to the promotion of risk-reducing behaviors, HIV testing for those who are at risk, and the facilitation of HIV services to those who have already become infected. Open discussion of these taboo topics must especially be encouraged in API families and schools if we are to reach the next generation of young Asian and Pacific Islanders before they become sexually active. We as educators need to take advantage of the fact that API youths become sexually active later than other ethnic groups, for it gives us time to educate them further and build stronger interpersonal communication skills concerning HIV related information. It is only through open communication that Asian and Pacific Islanders may halt the spread of AIDS within their communities and change perceptions of those already infected by the disease.

Issues Related to Sexuality.   Related to communication are the negative beliefs and attitudes concerning homosexuality and the resultant homophobia by some of the Asian community. These result in lack of communication between the infected person and healthcare providers as well as with family members who comprise the primary support group. One goal in health education and promotion is to enable the individual to view himself or herself as a human with healthcare needs similar to everyone else so as not to limit opportunities for obtaining the necessary counseling and guidance that can be offered by a qualified provider. One way this problem can be resolved is through the use of interactive computers. Paperny (1997) has shown that the candid nature of the computer which offers immediate, personalized feedback attracted adolescents to divulge sensitive information about their sexual history without the risk of destroying their anonymity and confidentiality. Therefore, when the provider learns that his client is gay, appropriate medical and support services can be offered when the individual needs them.

Heterosexuals and healthcare providers also must be encouraged to talk about their feelings with regard to homosexuality. This is very challenging, since homophobia is a deeply rooted part of cultural norms and mores. Parents may blame themselves for their child's homosexuality, regarding it as some kind of illness, or moral deviance. These behaviors and attitudes may span many generations. More important, heterosexual Asians need support in understanding the similarities they share with homosexuals in terms of needing to be loved, accepted, and recognized in their communities for the positive contributions they make to society. Therefore, educational material geared toward helping Asians understand the social obstacles of gay and lesbian Asians can lead to greater compassion toward all people with AIDS, regardless of their ethnicity.

Networking/Support Groups. Asian Americans participating in some form of support groups specific to their own ethnicity or gender issues may gain a deeper sense of belonging and identity. Networking reinforces the axiom that "there is strength in numbers" especially if members adhere to certain culture-specific protocols, such as speaking in the mother tongue only. Support groups that enforce culture-specific ways of interaction not only promote membership among recent immigrants who may still be experiencing culture shock, but also instill pride in their cultural heritage as well as support their sexual orientation. More important, support groups offer gay and lesbian Asians opportunities to gather in a safe social setting. For example, the gay Vietnamese friendship network in Los Angeles provides opportunities for Vietnamese gays and their partners to interact in an informal social setting. Membership to this group allows individuals to feel the support needed to deal with their sexual orientation, the homophobia in the Vietnamese community, loneliness, and isolation (Carrier, Nguyen, & Su, 1992). Networking with other gays, therefore, allows an individual to confront these issues without feeling that he is battling them alone.

Training of Healthcare Providers.   The same kind of moral and emotional support can be afforded by qualified health providers. However, problems occur when there are cultural clashes between therapist and client and are compounded by language and ethnicity differences. Although there is limited literature discussing the effect of therapist language and ethnicity and client outcomes, few studies appear to support a positive correlation between them (Flaskerud & Liu, 1990, 1991). Therefore, supportive services for Asians may include having a same-ethnicity therapist who is well versed in the client's language and culture. At the same time, the therapist must be willing to provide unconditional support through nonjudgmental ways of communicating. The therapist also must be patient and understand that issues related to someone's coming out or being gay, shame and guilt surrounding the disease, and unsafe sexual practices may be guarded privately by the client, and it may take time for the individual to honestly and openly discuss them.

Training of culturally competent and compassionate healthcare providers is imperative for Asians who are already reticent in discussing sexually related problems. Because of Asians' delay to seek treatment, healthcare providers should be astute in assessment and recognition of early signs and symptoms and risk behaviors relative to HIV infection. They should be assertive in a culturally sensitive manner when asking questions, making recommendations, and giving referrals.

Risk Behaviors.   How does one convince a certain population to stop engaging in unsafe sexual practices? This appears to be a major challenge confronting health providers and educators catering to Asians. Studies by Choi et al. (1995) have shown that API gay men tended to practice unprotected anal sex after engaging in substance use. The potent combination of these risky behaviors magnifies risk for acquiring AIDS. More alarming is the finding that many of these gay men maintain erroneous beliefs that they are not at risk for HIV despite their propensity to unsafe sex.

Understanding knowledge, beliefs, and attitudes about HIV/AIDS can be traced to the concept of collectivism. It is believed that because AIDS still is not as widespread among the Asian American community as in other racial groups, it is regarded as a nonthreat to them individually. It implies that people operate on some form of false bravado and continue to practice unsafe sex despite the overwhelming presence of AIDS in the community. Education and treatment programs need to convey the effects of AIDS on everyone.

Research Directions

Besides the studies on drug response and the incidence of tuberculosis and other AIDS-defining conditions, and the study on effectiveness of group counseling on risk behaviors, there are virtually no research studies on Asian Americans. One current study (Inouye & Oneha, 1997) investigating the use of self-management treatment strategies with Asian and Pacific Islanders has had difficulty in recruitment of subjects because of some of the previously identified barriers.

Now that some of the groundwork has been laid regarding attitudes, beliefs, and behaviors, the focus should move to determine the effective prevention programs, the effects of HIV infection on the Asian American community, and the differential responses to treatment and outcomes of this disease. Important prevention topics should include (a) the development of culturally competent health promotion and prevention strategies; (b) culturally sensitive education methods addressing different vulnerable subgroups and genders; (c) effectiveness of training methods of cultural competence in healthcare professionals to increase their communication and counseling skills in early identification and assessment; (d) investigation of the effectiveness of public relations and mass media campaigns targeting Asian Americans; and (e) attitudes, fears, and public policy issues concerning testing and treatment.

Intervention or treatment topics for research should include (a) utilization of alternative and complementary therapies in conjunction with or independent of allopathic healthcare and their effects on symptoms (some of which are currently under investigation) (Zhang & Ziolkowski, 1990); (b) training and support of family as caretakers; (c) the effects of expansion of ethnic resources in the community on healthcare utilization and prevention of secondary symptoms; (d) expansion of studies on different coping issues—adaptive and maladaptive—affecting Asian Americans; (e) the effects of culturally competent psychotherapy on levels of psychological distress; and (f) differential therapy outcome research specific for Asian Americans.

CONCLUSION

While the incidence of HIV/AIDS is low in the Asian American community, the group is at a precipice of risk for this epidemic. We have seen the difficulties involved in working with the Asian American community. They include vastly different, contradictory at times, behaviors, attitudes, and beliefs from the Western viewpoint. The communication difficulties—both linguistically and culturally—have resulted in a lack of understanding the many facets of the disease and its treatment. Reticence in discussion of areas related to sexuality and stoicism in relation to early healthcare operate to make difficult the task of education and health promotion. The challenges are many but knowledge, information, and dedicated professionals are available to overcome these in providing culturally competent care for this emerging group.

REFERENCES

AIDS Community Care Team and the Governor's Committee on HIV/AIDS. (1996, December). *HIV and AIDS in Hawaii: Status report and policy statement.* Honolulu, HI.

Albrecht, G. L., Levy, J. A., Sugrue, N. M., Proshaska, T. R., & Ostrow, D. G. (1989). Who hasn't heard about AIDS? *AIDS Education and Prevention, 1,* 261–267.

Aoki, B., Ngin, C., Mo, B., & Ja, D. (1989). Aids prevention models in Asian-American communities. *American Journal of Public Health, 79,* 448–452.

Brown, W. J. (1992). Culture and AIDS education: Reaching high-risk heterosexuals in Asian-American communities. *Journal of Applied Communication Research,* 275–291.

Carrier, J., Nguyen, B., & Su, S. (1992). Vietnamese American sexual behaviors & HIV infection. *Journal of Sex Research, 29*(4), 547–560.

Centers for Disease Control and Prevention. (1994). U.S. AIDS cases reported through December 1993. *HIV/AIDS surveillance report* (pp. 1–33). Atlanta, GA: Author.

Centers for Disease Control and Prevention. (1995). Update: Trends in AIDS among men who have sex with men—United States: 1989-1994. *MMWR Morbidity and Mortality Weekly Report, 44,* 401–404.

Choi, K. H., Lew, S., Vittinghoff, E., Catania, J. A., Barrett, D. C., & Coates, T. J. (1996). The efficacy of brief group counseling in HIV risk reduction among homosexual Asian and Pacific Islanders. *AIDS, 10,* 81–87.

Choi, K. H., Salazar, N., Lew, S., & Coates, T. J. (1995). AIDS risk, dual identity, and community response among gay Asian and Pacific Islander men in the United States. In G. M. Herek & B. Green (Eds.), *AIDS, identity, and community: The HIV epidemic and lesbians and gay men* (pp. 115–134). Thousand Oaks: Sage.

Cochran, S. D., Mays, V. M., & Leung, L. (1991). Sexual practices of heterosexual Asian-American young adults: Implications for risk of HIV infection. *Archives of Sexual Behavior, 20*(4), 381–391.

County of San Diego. (1994). *Description of the epidemic*. San Diego, CA: Department of Health Services, County of San Diego.

DiClemente, R. J., Zorn, J., & Temoshok, L. (1987). The association of gender, ethnicity, and length of residence in the Bay area to adolescents' knowledge and attitudes about Acquired Immune Deficiency Syndrome. *Journal of Applied Social Psychology, 17,* 216–230.

Eckholdt, H., Chin, J., Manzon, J., & Kim, D. (1994). Challenges of addressing needs of Asian and Pacific Islanders living with HIV in New York City. *International Conference on AIDS, 10,* 363. (Abstract No. PD0060)

Ekstrand, M., & Coates, T. J. (1990). Maintenance of safer sexual behaviors and predictors of risky sex: The San Francisco men's health study. *American Journal of Public Health, 80,* 973–977.

Flaskerud, J. H., & Liu, P. Y. (1990). Influence of therapist ethnicity and language on therapy outcomes of Southeast Asian clients. *International Journal of Social Psychiatry, 36*(1), 18–29.

Flaskerud, J. H., & Liu, P. Y. (1991). Effects of an Asian client-therapist language, ethnicity and gender match on utilization and outcome of therapy. *Community Mental Health Journal, 27*(1), 31–42.

Flaskerud, J. H., & Nyamathi, A. M. (1988, December). An AIDS education program for Vietnamese women. *New York State Journal of Medicine,* 632–637.

Gellert, G. A., Maxwell, R. M., Higgins, K. V., Mai, K. K., Lowery, R., & Doll, L. (1995). HIV/AIDS knowledge and high risk sexual practices among southern California Vietnamese. *Genitourinary Medicine, 71,* 216–223.

Gellert, G. A., Moore, D. F., Maxwell, R. M., Mai, K. K., & Higgins, K. V. (1994). Targeted HIV seroprevalence among Vietnamese in southern California. *Genitourinary Medicine, 70,* 265–267.

Gibaldi, M. (1993). Ethnic differences in the assessment and treatment of disease. *Pharmacotherapy, 13*(3), 170–176.

Gock, T. S. (1994). Acquired immunodeficiency syndrome. In N. Zane, D. Takeuchi, & K. Young (Eds.), *Confronting critical health issues of Asian and Asian and Pacific Islander Americans* (pp. 247–265). Thousand Oaks, CA: Sage.

Goh, D. S. (1993). Effects of HIV/AIDS information on attitudes toward AIDS: A cross-ethnic comparison of college students. *Journal of Psychology, 127*(6), 611–618.

Hirayama, H., & Hirayama, K. K. (1986). The sexuality of Japanese Americans. *Journal of Social Work and Human Sexuality, 4*(3), 81–98.

Hofstede, G. (1984). Hofstede's culture dimensions: An independent validation using Rokeach's value survey. *Journal of Cross-Cultural Psychology, 15,* 417–433.

Horan, P. F., & DiClemente, R. J. (1993). HIV knowledge, communication, and risk behaviors among White, Chinese-, and Filipino-American adolescents in a high-prevalence AIDS epicenter: A comparative analysis. *Ethnicity and Disease, 3,* 97–105.

Inouye, J., & Oneha, M. (1997). Patterns of health and illness in people living with HIV/AIDS. *Communicating Nursing Research, 30*(5), 75.

Ja, D. Y., & Ngin, P. (1987). *AIDS in the Asian community: A review and analysis.* Unpublished manuscript.

Jew, S. (1991). AIDS among California Asian and Pacific Islander subgroups. *California HIV/AIDS Update, 4*(9), 90-98.

Kitano, K. (1988). *Correlates of AIDS-associated high-risk behavior among Chinese and Filipino gay men.* Master's thesis, University of California, Berkeley.

Lin-Fu, J. S. (1993). Asian and Pacific Islander Americans: an overview of demographic characteristics and health care issues. *Asian American and Pacific Islander Journal of Health, Inaugural Issue 1*(1), 20-60.

Loue, S., Lloyd, L., & Loh, L. (1996). HIV prevention in U.S. Asian Pacific Islander communities: An innovative approach. *Journal of Health Care for the Poor and Underserved, 7*(4), 364-376.

Loue, S., Lloyd, L., & Phoombour, E. (1994). Beliefs about HIV among Asian/Pacific Islanders. *International Conference on AIDS, 10*(1), 361. (Abstract No. PD0049)

Metler, R., Hu, D. J., Fleming, P. L., & Ward, J. W. (1994). AIDS among Asian and Pacific Islanders (A/PI) reported in the USA. *International Conference on AIDS, 10*(2), 241. (Abstract No. PC0325)

Moore, D. S., & Erikson, P. I. (1985). Age, gender, and ethnic differences in sexual and contraceptive knowledge, attitudes, and behaviors. *Family Community Health, 8,* 38-51.

National AIDS Network. (1989). The many faces of Asian AIDS. *NAN Multi-Cultural Notes on AIDS Education and Services, 2*(3), 1-2.

Osmond, D. H., Page, K., Wiley, J., Garrett, K., Sheppard, H. W., Moss, A. R., Schrager, L., & Winkelstein, W. (1994). HIV infection in homosexual and bisexual men 18 to 29 years of age: The San Francisco young men's health study. *American Journal of Public Health, 84,* 1933-1937.

Paperny, D. M. (1997). Computerized health assessment and education for adolescent HIV and STD prevention in health care settings and schools. *Health Education & Behavior, 24*(1), 54-70.

Prohaska, T. R., Albrecht, G., Levy, J. A., Sugrue, N., & Kim, J. H. (1990). Determinants of self-perceived risk for AIDS. *Journal of Health and Social Behavior, 31,* 384-394.

Sidhu, J. S., Weinstock, H., & Gwinn, M. (1996). HIV seroprevalence among Asian/Pacific Islanders attending sexually transmitted disease clinics in the United States, 1989-1994. *International Conference on AIDS, 11*(1), 128. (Abstract No. Mo.C.1421)

State of Hawaii. (1997). *AIDS Surveillance Quarter Reports.* Honolulu, HI.

Strunin, L. (1991). Adolescents' perceptions of risk for HIV infection: Implications for future research. *Social Science Medicine, 32*(2), 221-228.

Studemeister, A. E., & Kent, G. P. (1993). Prevalence of Human Immunodeficiency Virus infection in a sample of immigrants in the United States. *Western Journal of Medicine, 158,* 145-147.

Swanson, G. M., & Ward, A. J. (1995). Recruiting minorities into clinical trials: Toward a participant friendly system. *Journal of the National Cancer Institute, 87*(23), 1747-1759.

Toleran, D. E. (1991). Pakikisama: Reaching the Filipino community with AIDS prevention. *Multicultural Inquiry Res AIDS Q Newsletter, 5*(1), 8-10.

U.S. Bureau of the Census. (1992). *Population projections of the United States, by age, sex, race, and Hispanic origin: 1992 to 2050* (P. 25-2092). Washington DC: U.S. Government Printing Office.

Woo, J. M., Rutherford, G. W., Payne, S. F., Barnhart, J. L., & Lemp, G. F. (1988). The epidemiology of AIDS in Asian and Pacific Islander populations in San Francisco. *AIDS, 2,* 473-475.

Workgroup on Health Care Access Issues for Asian and Pacific Islanders. (1994). *HIV/AIDS.* Health Resources and Services Administration: Washington, DC.

Yep, G. A. (1992-93). HIV/AIDS in Asian and Pacific Islander communities in the U.S.: A review, analysis, and integration. *International Quarterly of Community Health Education, 13*(4), 293-315.

Yep, G. A. (1993a). First Asian/Pacific Island Men's HIV Conference, Los Angeles, California. *AIDS Education and Prevention, 5*(1), 87-88.

Yep, G. A. (1993b). HIV prevention among Asian-American college students: Does the Health Belief Model work? *Journal of American College Health, 41*(5) 199-205.

Yep, G. A. (1994). HIV/AIDS education and prevention for Asian and Pacific Islander communities: Toward the development of general guidelines. *AIDS Education and Prevention, 6*(2), 184-186.

Yoshioka, M. R., Chin, J., & Manzon, J. A. (1996). Asian and Pacific Islanders living with HIV/AIDS in New York City: In search of cultural competence. *International Conference on AIDS, 11*(1), 207. (Abstract No. Mo.D. 1908)

Zhang, Q., & Ziolkowski, H. (1990). Treating HIV disease with Chinese medicine. *Focus: A guide to AIDS Research and Counseling, 5*(10), 1-2.

CHAPTER EIGHT

Buddhist Ethics and Implications for End-of-Life Issues

Ide Pang Katims, PhD, RN

*F*or over two thousand years, Buddhism has been a strong influencing force in every Asian society. It deeply affects the ways in which people view their world and decide on what is important in their personal, family, and community lives.

Buddhism has also taken firm roots in Europe and the United States. Healthcare professionals must consider Buddhist ethics as an additional framework for ethical decision making. Buddhism casts a different light on contemporary problems that have resulted from the use of medical technology; the competing interest between oneself, family, and the community; as well as many other critical and urgent questions relating to healthcare.

This chapter describes beliefs and concepts fundamental to Buddhism and Buddhist ethics. The moral framework of Buddhist ethics is to analyze issues surrounding end-of-life care; specifically, a definition of death acceptable to Buddhism, related responses to the care of individuals in persistent vegetative state, and euthanasia.

Buddhism is a body of religious teachings attributed to a historical individual who lived in northeast India during the fifth century B.C., and who became known as "Buddha," or "enlightened one." Buddha claimed no divine knowledge, but presented his teachings as immutable laws expressing the natural and moral order of things. As those teachings spread throughout Asia, each took on distinctive characteristics and unique emphases in India, Tibet, China, Japan, and southeast Asia.

BELIEFS AND CONCEPTS FUNDAMENTAL TO BUDDHISM

Despite the cultural stamps on the Buddhist teachings, some basic principles and beliefs remain consistent throughout the world. Personal realization and spiritual transformation are believed to be brought about by living in accordance with Buddha's teachings, the cornerstones of which are the Four Noble Truths. These maintain that (a) life as we know it is imperfect and unsatisfactory, unsatisfactory because of people's craving and ignorance; (b) there exists a state of perfect freedom from life's unsatisfactoriness; and (c) the way to perfect freedom is the Eightfold Path, which is a prescription for right living, moral cultivation, meditation, and knowledge of the human condition.

Morality is part of the spiritual journey that cultivates a wholesome character (e.g., by refraining from stealing or taking life). Together with meditation and awareness of the human condition, a gradual personal transformation becomes possible and culminates in Nirvana, a state of liberation from all traces of greed, attachment, hatred, delusion, and their consequent sufferings. Such a vision assumes that people have no fixed, unchanging "self." Each person is capable of radical transformation brought about by attention to the nature of mind and action.

Although precepts by which a person can live a wholesome life are readily available, Buddhism offers no carefully constructed theoretical formulation to explain its assumptions and prescriptions. Within the contemporary Western approach to Buddhism, however, there does exist a desire to articulate a clear moral structure so that the "ethics" grounded in Buddhist teachings can be more useful in the Western ethics milieu. To this end, attempts have been made to retrofit Buddhism with Western theoretical frameworks including William James' pragmatism (Kalupahana, 1988) and Christian social ethics (Ives, 1992). Keown (1992, 1995) has also drawn careful parallels between Buddhism and Aristotelian natural law, and together with Whitehill (1987, 1994), suggested that Buddhism can be viewed as a "virtue ethic," in line with philosophers such as MacIntyre (1984) and Hauerwas (1981). This cross-cultural dialogue has certainly enriched Western attentiveness to Buddhism as a whole, making its belief system less mysterious and more usable in ethical decision making.

In many ways, no fixed set of behaviors can be labeled as precisely ethical behaviors in Buddhism. The central premise of Buddhist ethical life involves an awareness of interdependence, out of which emerges compassion. This is a particularly prominent concept in the Buddhist tradition of Japan and Korea, where the "emptiness theory" is emphasized.

Here, the isolated self, or "I," is cast aside for the interconnected tie we have with all things around us. Compassion is, in one sense, a personal goal, but by definition also extends outward from the individual as a transformative openness to the world. Together with other Buddhist virtues, such as respect for life and knowledge of the natural order of things, this awareness helped to create a strong moral foundation for and across Asian societies.

Buddhism originated as a movement to renounce social life, not to enmesh in its problems. Thus it had little to say about ethics, especially regarding concerns considered significant in the Western world, such as demands for human rights, individual autonomy, and privacy. Nonetheless, Buddhism's benevolent and humane moral values are widely respected. In this light, the Buddhist notion of compassion is closely akin to the growing realization that people, communities, and societies are interdependent, and to the caring values promulgated by health care professionals. Ultimately, some formal examination of Buddhist teaching for ethical decision making has become necessary by virtue of the social and cultural fact of diversity and the need for nurses, physicians, and other healthcare providers to give culturally competent care. More specifically for this discussion, it is no longer adequate to rely solely on frameworks of Western medical ethics to help individuals and families of Buddhist orientations confront and make choices about issues related to end-of-life care.

CONTRASTING WESTERN AND BUDDHIST VIEWS OF PERSONHOOD

Prior to discussing the values related to end-of-life choices, it is important to reflect upon what it means to be a person during a lifetime. Personhood is a central problem for both Western medical ethics and Buddhist ethics, but these two traditions differ significantly in how a person is viewed.

For Western medical ethics, a representative definition of a person is someone who is "rational, is capable of free choices, and is a coherent, continuing and autonomous center of sensations, experiences, emotions, volitions, and actions" (Mahoney, 1984, p. 54). American philosopher Josiah Royce indicated that people generally and characteristically assert:

> *We are beings, each of whom has a soul of his own, a destiny of his own, rights of his own, worth of his own, ideals of his own, and an individual*

life in which this soul, this destiny, these rights, these ideals, get their ex-
pression. No other man can do my deed for me. When I choose, my choice
coalesces with the voluntary decision of no other individual. (Fisch,
1951, p. 202)

What makes a human being worthy of the moral status of person—with
all its attendant dignity and respect—is the autonomous self and its capacity to act with a free will. From this standpoint, having the ability to control personal destiny and lifestyle, living an acceptable quality of life, and
possessing the capacity for self-determination are of critical importance.
Loss of control, the inability to perceive sensations, experiences and emotions, in contrast, certainly undermine the status of person and may even
make life not worth living. In this regard, while all persons are human beings, not all human beings are persons. For example, a fetus in the early
stages of development lacks many elements of personhood. Prior to birth in
the early stages of life, the biological material is, at best, a potential person.
The same is true of an adult with severe dementia. He or she is no longer a
"person," because many of the capacities that are deemed essential in
being "person" are absent or lost.

Whether overtly or covertly, Americans have been arguing about euthanasia and removal from life support of individuals in persistent vegetative state for decades. While such arguments are often contextualized
within issues pertaining to privacy—that is, seeking to end one's life is
posed as an intimate, personal matter—the real points at issue are control
of one's destiny and the belief that quality of life may be more important
than life itself.

Buddhists present a very different view of human nature. While all attributes of personhood such as rationality, volition, and ability to make
choices and take action are acknowledged to exist, the human being is regarded as a complex of mental and biological elements with a history and
destiny that transcend a single lifetime. When a person dies, he or she undergoes rebirth and returns to the living. From this standpoint, human existence is a continuum with a long biography which represents the same
being or development of that being over many lifetimes. Individual lives
thus form different episodes in a person's continuous biography. Whatever the circumstances of life, his or her moral status remains unchanged.
There are no unique markers of human nature, such as rationality and autonomy, that provide a basis for a person's moral status. Instead, the Buddhist "person" represents a psycho-physical totality of the human being
along an individual evolutionary trajectory.

When viewed in the context of rebirth and continuity, the concept of personhood, even the notion of "I" or "self" become quite irrelevant. With no substantial and permanent self or I, self-centered human actions (rooted in the I-view or I-attitude) are out of sync with Buddhist reality. As a result, the need to control one's everyday domain becomes less acute. With the intuitive understand that one is part of a larger universe that includes all living beings in past and future lives, death is no longer feared as a terrible finality.

ETHICAL BELIEFS IN BUDDHISM

In the absence of a systematic theory of ethics in Buddhism, what, then, is its vision of human good? For Keown (1995), three basic goods are clearly identifiable: life, wisdom, and compassion.

Buddhism expresses profound respect for life, especially life that possesses a moral biography and undergoes rebirth. All life forms are believed to have existed in their respective evolutionary trajectories—insects, animals, demons, and human beings (Kapleau, 1980). Thus, noninjury to human beings and animals is a distinguishing mark of Buddhist teaching. At the same time, treating illnesses by means of the healing arts becomes a moral action by virtue of its life-preserving intent. Such respect for life, however, does not mean that life must be preserved at all cost.

Wisdom develops out of knowing Buddhist doctrine and having the opportunity to transcend the limitations imposed by human ignorance and selfishness which also allows for the fulfillment of one's natural abilities. Knowledge of Buddhist doctrine and consideration of how to live by its precepts are viewed as intrinsically good. Buddhism also maintains that the truth about right and wrong can be objectively known through proper use of the intellectual faculties.

Again according to Keown (1995), the concept of compassion in Buddhism has two meanings: the inclination to empathize with the suffering of others and compassion, a totality of moral virtues an enlightened person would possess—benevolence, generosity, rejoicing in others' good fortunes, patience, tolerance, and friendship.

For a Buddhist, the general rules of action as expressed in everyday life aim at supporting the three basic goods. These precepts admonish people to refrain from certain kinds of acts, with the taking of life as one of the most serious infractions. These precepts also may be viewed as norms imposed upon people so that certain values are protected and promoted. Some rules inculcate restraint and self-discipline; others regulate community life. For example, there are the five precepts for laymen, which forbid taking life, stealing, sexual misconduct, lying, and taking intoxicants. The values themselves are not necessarily moral values, but the issue of morality arises when choices are made with respect to them.

BUDDHISM AND DEATH

In Buddhism's holistic understanding of nature, everything is part of the larger process of birth and decay, through which things come into being and then pass away: day turns into night, monuments turn into rubble, the human body turns into dust. Although human death is part of this larger process, a survivor's grief is no less real or intense. In fact, old age and death are two aspects of suffering that appear often in Buddhist stories. It is the development of insight into the ultimate unsustainability of material things, including the biological body, that brings acceptance and peace. The parable of the mustard seed offers such a lesson:

> *The Buddha was once approached by a woman half mad with grief over the death of her newborn child. Laying the baby at his feet, she pleaded with him to restore it to life. After listening patiently the Buddha told her to go into town and bring back a mustard seed from a house in which there had never been a death. The woman went from door to door throughout the entire city but found not a house untouched by death. Realizing that death comes to all, she finally accepted the fate of her child. (Kapleau, 1980, p. 158)*

Buddhist writings identified three factors that distinguish a living from a dead body: the presence of vitality, heat, and consciousness (Keown, 1995). Vitality and heat, according to Keown, are indicators of life and belong to the biological makeup of the person. Vitality may be viewed as the physical life force. Heat probably refers to the energy generated by the basic metabolic processes within a living body (Keown, 1995). The existence of vitality is believed to be dependent upon heat, and the human faculties of sight, hearing, smell, taste, and touch are, in turn, dependent upon vitality. At death as consciousness leaves the biological body, vitality and heat also dissipate. From the Buddhist perspective, death can be best described as biological in nature. Little emphasis is placed on the marks of personhood that distinguish Western views, such as the loss of rationality, awareness, and self-consciousness.

A Definition of Death Acceptable to Buddhist Ethics

Traditionally, the cessation of respiration and heartbeat brings death. Yet recent advances in medical technology, providing for the artificial maintenance of bodily functions, have altered the criteria for identifying death. The almost simultaneous cessation of respiration and heartbeat often does not occur; an important development here is the formulation of a criterion for defining death in terms of the cessation of all brain functions, or total brain death. Neocortical brain death, when only certain parts of the brain are damaged and there is irreversible loss of all higher brain functions, is commonly associated with people in the persistent vegetative state, and it also complicates the discussion.

Mettanando (1991) and Keown (1995) have argued that vitality, or human physical life force, as described in Buddhist texts, is credited with the coordination and integration of the basic organic processes that sustain life—much like the functions attributed to the human brainstem. Here, it seems, ancient Buddhist beliefs intersect with modern medicine. Mettanando and Keown conclude that if, from the Buddhist standpoint, vitality dissipates at death, then the Buddhist view of death is consistent with death of the brainstem: when all vital bodily functions are no longer coordinated by the brainstem.

Brainstem death is distinguishable from neocortical brain death. Mettanando points out that the latter is total cessation of physical functions; however, the former is irreversible loss of only high-level consciousness— the brainstem remains intact and functioning, and spontaneous breathing and reflexes such as the dilation of the pupils are present. Wrongly called brain dead, people with irreversible loss of high-level brain functions are in what is known as persistent vegetative state. For Buddhism, the loss of higher brain functions does not render a person dead. Human beings are biological creatures; death must be a biological death, the criterion of which is the brain's inability to coordinate organic functioning of the body.

Persistent Vegetative State.   Consider the case of Nancy Cruzan: For over seven years, Ms. Cruzan was in persistent vegetative state without cognitive brain function and felt no pain. Although she was able to breathe on her own (indicating a functioning brainstem), she received nutrition and fluids through a feeding tube inserted into her stomach. A legal battle ensued over whether Ms. Cruzan herself would have wished to terminate her life of permanent unconsciousness, and whether her family had the right to make that decision for her.

For Ms. Cruzan, it seems the value placed on her life diminished in relation to her loss of higher brain functions. As her life ceased to have any recognizable human value, her existence lost its meaning. With that, the Cruzan family and many others argued that Ms. Cruzan's life was not worth living and concluded that she should have the right to die. To exercise this right, the Cruzan family asked to have the feeding tube removed.

With Buddhism's deep respect for life, it would be morally wrong to bring about the death of an individual in persistent vegetative state by withholding food and fluids. Causing another person to die by starvation and dehydration yields weighty consequences, a process known as "karma" in Buddhist terminology. Karma, or law of causality in moral experience, teaches that wholesome actions bring about good consequences. Unwholesome acts, such as taking a human life, impose long-term, serious retribution; for example, rebirth into a lower form of animal life, or the prospect of future lives filled with great pain and suffering.

As such, in the case of persistent vegetative state, patients who have not been declared dead by the criteria of brainstem death should not be made to suffer the withholding of food and hydration. At the same time, in Buddhist ethics there is no requisite for extraordinary measures to preserve life at all costs, such as using life support machines simply to keep patients alive. After all, life and death are merely part of the larger process of birth and decay. If persistent vegetative state is the final phase of the dying process, death will come at its conclusion at the appropriate time.

Humane and ethical care for such patients is consistent with the Buddhist virtue of compassion. All persons, regardless of physical condition, are worthy of compassionate concern. The total care needed by people in persistent vegetative state, in fact, affords caregivers the opportunity to cultivate the many moral virtues associated with compassion, such as empathy, benevolence, patience, and affirmation of friendship and human bonds.

Euthanasia

Euthanasia is defined as the act of causing death for reasons of mercy. In the context of medical care, euthanasia is "the intentional killing of a patient by act or omission as part of his [or her] medical care" (Keown, 1995, p. 168). To distinguish euthanasia from situations in which patients refuse medical treatment to their own detriment, an essential character- istic of all forms of euthanasia is that the death of the patient is directly willed by the person who either acts or omits to act with the intention of causing the patient's death.

There are active and passive modes of euthanasia. Active euthanasia is the deliberate killing of a patient by lethal injection or other means. Passive euthanasia is the intentional causing of death by an omission; withholding food and fluids, for example. While the American Medical Association (AMA) opposes active euthanasia, it finds passive euthanasia morally per- missible (Bandman & Bandman, 1990). In the Western ethical milieu, pas- sive euthanasia may even be viewed as a compassionate act when patients, stating personal freedom and autonomy, plea with their physicians to let them die. They have determined that life with a terminal illness and pain is not worth living.

From the perspective of Buddhist ethics, euthanasia is never permissi- ble. The first and most significant Buddhist precept prohibits killing, even when the person being killed requests assistance in dying. Any course of action involving an intentional choice against life is deemed wrongful because by doing so, life is denied as a basic good. Moreover, human life is supremely precious in Buddhism: It is only from this state that a person can realize enlightenment and free him- or herself from the unending suffering of many lifetimes of birth, death, and rebirth. This be- lief is central to the morality of Buddhism.

Kapleau (1989) has offered the perspective that euthanasia is not a means of escape from suffering and pain. "Buddhism holds that because death is not the end, suffering does not cease thereupon, but continues until the karma that created the suffering has played itself out; thus it is pointless to kill oneself—or aid another to do so—in order to escape" (p. 135). Furthermore, Lecso (1996) suggested that "in Buddhism a termi- nal illness is not considered a chance event . . . a terminal illness represents the repayment of a karmic debt" (p. 55). By disrupting the course of karma, one merely pushes the pain and suffering of this lifetime into future life- times. Kapleau (1980) also has proposed that those sufferers who under- stand the meaning of pain and its relation to karma—that is, the grateful acceptance of pain as a means of paying karmic debts—would not ask for euthanasia.

If there is an alternative that Buddhist ethics offer to euthanasia, it is this: Even if people live out the pain of terminal illness, nothing precludes them from receiving humanistic and compassionate palliative care, with an aim toward relieving physical discomfort and mental distress.

IMPLICATIONS FOR HEALTHCARE PROVIDERS

The moral framework of Buddhist ethics demands a holistic, humanistic, and organic view of life and death. The Buddhist belief in the interdependence of things—a theme of prominence in Buddhist teachings—alerts healthcare providers to the need for a different approach when working with patients and families holding Buddhist orientations. No longer adequate is the sole reliance on theories from Western medical ethics that feature the autonomous, self-determining moral agent. Ethical decision-making guidelines framed from the perspective of Buddhist ethics provide a viable alternative as our cultural society becomes increasingly diverse, and where nurses, physicians, and other healthcare providers are morally obligated to provide culturally competent care.

Some understanding of Buddhist cosmology, such as the notions of rebirth and karma, would help healthcare providers form a more genuine and empathic bond with patients of Asian heritage. When these patients fail to accept a recommendation that, to the mind of the healthcare provider, is clearly beneficial, as for example, when a patient with terminal illness and intractable pain refuses to take pain medication because he or she claims that it clouds the mind, the healthcare provider needs to know that the person may not be irrational or lacking the capacity to make decisions to protect him- or herself. Rather, he or she simply may be accepting the physical pain as a karmic debt, and counting on clarity of mind, unhindered by medication, to gain insight and wisdom during the dying process.

It must be kept in mind, however, that not all people of Asian heritage practice Buddhism. For those who do, the majority are neither enlightened, nor are they thoroughly ignorant of the Buddhist precepts for a wholesome life. Most people live a practical life, which is an interplay of increasing awareness set against karmic backsliding. For people of Asian heritage, the popular expressions of Buddhist virtues are often neither religious nor philosophical, but thoroughly integrated into the value system of family and community relationships. Thus the Buddhist worldview and values may be more prevalent in people's habits of thinking then they themselves are aware. It is therefore critical that healthcare providers are knowledgeable about this alternative worldview, especially as it relates to end-of-life issues.

REFERENCES

Bandman, E. L., & Bandman, B. (1990). *Nursing ethics through the life span.* East Norwalk, CT: Appleton & Lange.

Fisch, M. H. (Ed.). (1951). *Classic American philosophers.* New York: Appleton-Century-Crofts.

Hauerwas, S. (1981). *A community of character.* Notre Dame, IN: University of Notre Dame Press.

Ives, C. A. (1992). *Zen awakening and society.* Honolulu: University of Hawaii Press.

Kalupahana, D. J. (1988, July). The buddhist conceptions of "subject" and "object" and their moral implications. *Philosophy East and West, 33,* 290–304.

Kapleau, P. (1980). *Zen: Dawn in the West.* New York: Anchor Press.

Kapleau, P. (1989). *The wheel of life and death.* New York: Doubleday.

Keown, D. (1992). *The nature of buddhist ethics.* New York: St. Martin Press.

Keown, D. (1995). *Buddhism and bioethics.* New York: St. Martin Press.

Lecso, P. A. (1996). Euthanasia: A Buddhist perspective. *Journal of Religion and Health, 25,* 51-57.

MacIntyre, A. (1984). *After virtue.* Notre Dame, IN: University of Notre Dame Press.

Mahoney, J. (1984). *Bioethics and belief.* London: Sheed and Ward.

Mettanando, B. (1991). Buddhist ethics in the practice of medicine. In C. W. Fu & S. A. Wawrytkoin (Eds.), *Buddhist ethics and modern society: An international symposium* (pp. 195–213). New York: Greenwood Press.

Whitehill, J. (1987). Is there a Zen ethic? *The Eastern Buddhist (New Series) 20,* 9-33.

Whitehill, J. (1994). Buddhist ethics in western context: The virtues approach. *Journal of Buddhist Ethics,* 1-22.

CHAPTER NINE

The Dilemma in Searching for Healthcare: The Scenario of Chinese American Elderly Immigrants

Zibin Guo, Ph.D.

*H*ealthcare seeking behavior is a complex phenomenon. This is espe-cially true when dealing with elderly immigration populations whose cultural traditions, health culture, and healthcare system in their soci-eties of origin differ from those in the society in which they currently live. In such a case, the relationship between individuals' healthcare seek-ing behavior and the factors that generate the behavior become even more complicated.

Retrospectively, there has been no lack of research literature regarding health and healthcare of elderly Asian Americans, especially the Chinese elderly population. Studies demonstrate that elderly Chinese are extraordi-narily vulnerable in American society (Carp & Kataoka, 1976; P. Chen, 1979; Cheng, 1978; M. Cheung, 1989; Lum & Cheung, 1980; E. Wong, 1980; Wu, 1975; Ying, 1985; Yu, 1981, 1983, 1984). The language barrier, lack of knowledge about American society and its healthcare system, differ-ent cultural assumptions about health and illness, cultural stereotypes, intergenerational conflict, and discrimination by people in the health-care system, all are factors that play a role in preventing elderly Chinese from receiving proper health and social services (V. Chen, 1989; Fujii, 1976; Ikels, 1983; Liu, 1986; Nagasawa, 1980; Yu, 1983). For many of these elderly, when healthcare was needed, traditional Chinese medicine practitioners provided the few available services to them (Hessler et al., 1975). Studies suggest that one reason many elderly individuals remain in

Chinese communities is that they can obtain Chinese healthcare practitioners (P. Chen, 1979; M. Cheung, 1989; B. Wong, 1982).

The purpose of this chapter is not to evaluate the effectiveness of the programs and policies aimed to change and improve elderly Asian Americans' healthcare conditions. Rather, it is to focus on a recently immigrated Chinese elderly population in King City (pseudonym), a developing multicultural urban community in New York City. This chapter, through a mixture of qualitative and quantitative ethnographic techniques, examines interaction dynamics between elderly Chinese and modern healthcare services available to them, and the major factors affecting elderly Chinese immigrants' healthcare seeking behaviors and decision making.

KING CITY

King City is situated northeast of the New York City metropolitan area. Two decades ago, King City, which once had been a moderately prosperous suburban community, experienced a significant period of economic depression. At this time, while new settlers moved to the city, old settlers—middle-class White Americans in particular—moved away in search of opportunities. Alternatively, the economic depression and resulting decline of real estate values in the area created opportunities for the new settlers. A large number of recent immigrants moved into the area to re-create their former enclaves.

At the end of the 1970s, increasing numbers of Chinese, particularly Taiwanese, began moving into the King City area. Chinese restaurants, grocery stores, and other businesses were established. Soon families from the Indian subcontinent also moved into the area. Unlike earlier Asian immigrants, among the new arrivals was a large number of middle-class individuals who brought with them considerable financial assets. The arrival of these new settlers changed King City dramatically, a city once known as a "Sleeping dog."[1] By 1990, the community was a rapidly developing center of commercial activity, with large numbers of immigrants from Taiwan, mainland China, Korea, India, and other Asian populations.

Although the 1990 U.S. census identified 20,352 Chinese Americans in King City (see Table 9.1), among the informants and others involved in

---

[1] Richard Gelman, president of National Bank of New York City used the term "Sleeping dog" to refer to the old King City when talking to a reporter of *The Wall Street Journal* (in Wysocki, 1991).

Table 9.1   Population Change in King City (by Origin)

Origin	1980		1990		Change 1980–1990	
	Number	Percent	Number	Percent	Number	Percent
Eurp. Amer.	156,282	76.3	129,172	58.2	−27,110	−17.3
Afri. Amer.	9,580	4.7	9,352	4.2	−228	−2.4
Hispanic	20,045	9.8	33,299	15.0	13,254	66.1
Chinese	6,700	3.3	20,352	9.2	13,652	203.8
Asian Ind.	4,592	2.2	7,200	3.2	2,608	56.8
Korean	3,794	1.9	17,803	8.0	14,009	369.2
Filipino	919	0.4	1,909	0.9	990	107.7
Total Population	204,785	100.00	221,763	100.00	16,978	8.3

this research, no one is convinced of the accuracy of this figure. Most believe there are at least 40,000 to 50,000 Chinese living in King City.

Although it may be impossible to obtain precise data on the number of Chinese elderly in King City, according to interviews with community leaders and other sources, there are at least 3,000 elderly Chinese individuals in this multicultural community. This estimate is conservative when compared with the information discussed with the Department of City Planning (October 10, 1992), which states that senior citizens make up more than one-third of the total population in this community.

The Chinese elderly population in King City is heterogeneous. Its diversity is the result of variations in immigration patterns, diverse economic adaptations, and differing degrees of acculturation among the subgroups.

Taiwanese Immigrants

Elderly immigrants from Taiwan make up the largest subgroup of the Chinese elderly population in King City. Some of them are pioneers among Chinese immigrants to King City; however, most of these individuals immigrated in the past 15 years.

The majority of elderly individuals in this population are those who left mainland China for Taiwan at the end of the 1940s due to the end of the civil war between the Communists and the Guomindang Nationalists. Because of special circumstances present at the time, individuals who were able to withdraw from the mainland were mostly those associated with elite classes of the Guomindang government: military personnel, government officials, bureaucrats, businessmen, respected intellectuals and artists, and their family members. Most were Mandarin speaking. These Taiwan Mainlanders also can be divided into two main categories. Generally speaking, individuals in each are well educated and hail from well established urban families, with some having reached a high social status before emigrating.

Early Immigrants.   In the mid-1970s, as better relations between the United States and the People's Republic of China developed (especially after the two nations officially normalized their relations in 1979), many of these former Mainlanders began to leave Taiwan, finding their way to the United States. Their exodus occurred because of the concern that Taiwan would soon be attacked by the Communists from mainland China.

Later Immigrants.   The second movement of Taiwan-Mainlander immigration to the United States started in the late 1980s and early 1990s. During this period, as the independence movement among native Taiwanese developed, many of the aged former Mainlanders (who once comprised the dominant class) began to immigrate to the United States to avoid future political instability on the island.

Unlike the earlier immigrants, most of these individuals came to the States after reaching the age of retirement. Some came to the United States as business investors; others, to join their adult children who had previously come to receive an education and were now settled in the United States. Still others arrived under the sponsorship of relatives who had settled in the United States in earlier decades.

As Taiwan became one of the most economically successful areas in the world in the early 1980s, its standard of living became comparable with most of the well developed nations. The economic status of some Taiwan-Mainlander immigrants, especially among those who immigrated to this country within the past 10 years, generated a different lifestyle compared to other subgroups of the Chinese population in this community. Nationwide and worldwide tours are regularly organized by churches and senior groups for these individuals, and some also regularly travel to Taiwan and other destinations on their own.

Taiwan-Mainlanders in this community are not homogeneous in terms of socioeconomic status. Many elderly individuals of this subgroup continue working to earn a living, while others live on their social welfare benefits.

Mainland China Immigrants

Mainland China immigrants make up the second largest subgroup of Chinese Americans in King City. They can be further divided according to pattern and time of immigration.

CBS (Chinese-Born Students and Scholars).   This term is used to refer to Chinese elderly in King City who came to the United States from mainland China for an education or other endeavors, but due to World War II and the subsequent civil war in China, were unable to return to their homeland. Previously, some of them lived in non-Chinese communities, but because they desired to be close to their culture, they moved to King City for their retirement years.

New Immigrants.   The second type of mainland Chinese immigrants includes those who arrived during the past decade to join their children, many of whom came to the United States as students during the 1970s and 1980s, and who later settled in the King City area.

Included in this group were former intellectuals and administrators who suffered the various political movements of the 1950s and 1960s in mainland China. Some had strong educational backgrounds but little opportunity to advance socially and economically because family members were living in Taiwan or in the United States. A few, however, were able to elevate their status in mainland China.

Alternatively, since the end of the 1970s, the political climate has changed significantly, allowing most of these individuals to enjoy a moderate degree of social status in mainland China. Especially in the past 10 years, having a family member in either Taiwan or the United States became a social and political advantage for individual contacts. The reasons for immigration to the United States included familial and economic motives. And for some elderly Chinese, the major motivation was to bring their children to the United States.

Table 9.2, on the following page, illustrates the characteristics of surveyed Chinese American elderly in King City. Results show that the majority of surveyed individuals (86%) immigrated to the United States within the past 10 years. Large numbers of individuals from mainland China and Taiwan groups had high educational backgrounds. Thirty-one percent of the individuals were college graduates, 26% were high school graduates, and 17% were middle school graduates. Among those included, 65% reported that their previous occupation was either professional or business related.

Table 9.2   Characteristics of Surveyed Population

Gender
Male   39 (47%)
Female   44 (53%)

Age
60–69   43 (52%)
70–79   35 (42%)
80 and over   5   (6%)

Years in the United States
Within 5 years   52 (63%)
Within 10 years   19 (23%)
Within 15 years   12 (14%)

Education
Less than primary   14 (17%)
Primary   8   (9%)
Middle school   13 (17%)
High school   22 (26%)
College   26 (31%)

Occupation
Professional   9 (11%)
Business   45 (54%)
None prof.   14 (17%)
Other   15 (18%)

N = 83

HEALTHCARE SYSTEM WITHIN AND AROUND KING CITY

The healthcare system in King City is a complex pluralistic one, in which an ample number of established healthcare providers falls into three categories: Western-style and traditional Chinese practitioners and integrated healers.

Western-Style Healthcare Providers

The majority of healthcare providers in King City practice Western-style medicine. The Western-style system in King City is comprised of 2 private hospitals, about 200 private licensed Chinese physicians, over 50 nonlicensed Chinese physicians, and 5 Chinese-owned pharmacies.

The 200 licensed Chinese physicians represent 18 specialized areas from allergies to surgery (Chinese Business Directory, 1994). No doctor in this group specializes in geriatric medicine. Among the licensed physicians, 45 accept Medicare payments, yet only 3 accept Medicaid patients.

A large number of these physicians are American trained. They came from either Taiwan or Hong Kong in their younger years, received medical degrees, and settled in the United States. As more and more Chinese migrated to King City, physicians located to the area and established their medical practices. However, some are American-born Chinese physicians. The reasons that these individuals started their medical practices in King City include not only the increasing Chinese population, but also their ability to speak Mandarin.

Chinese Traditional Medicine Doctors

In order to get an inventory of Chinese traditional medicine practitioners in King City, I examined various sources such as local Chinese newspapers and magazines (in which many Chinese traditional medicine doctors advertised), as well as the newly published Chinese Business Directory. I found 74 Chinese traditional medicine doctors, of whom only 14 have either state or city acupuncture licenses. Since many do not want to publicize their services, the number of Chinese medical practitioners and healers listed in my sources may fall short of the actual total. Among the 15 Chinese traditional doctors I interviewed, only 4 of them advertise in the newspapers and directories.

Most of these traditional medicine practitioners claim to treat the full gamut of health problems, ranging from foot pain to stroke rehabilitation, from skin infections to heart disease. However, some advertise only specialized areas, such as body injury, arthritis, high blood pressure, lack of energy, hemorrhoids, anemia, kidney insufficiency, and calculosis.

Integrated Healers

The term *integrated medicine* was developed in mainland China four decades ago. It simply refers to the integration of traditional Chinese medicine (TCM) methods and those of Western medicine. In King City, at least five healthcare facilities advertise integrated practices. These facilities not only have attending physicians, but also sell herbs, Chinese-made Western drugs, and over-the-counter medications.

In one such facility I visited, there were three doctors: one a female who graduated from a Chinese traditional medicine college the previous year; a middle-age man who said he was an integrated doctor in China; and the third, a middle-age man who told me that he is good at Western medicine but likes Chinese traditional medicine methods as well. During one of my visits to this facility, this doctor explained:

> *Chinese traditional medicine is very good at treating disease, since it tends to get rid of the problem from its root, yet with minimal side effects. Western medicine has very advanced diagnosis technologies, but the drugs are too strong, and they often cause other problems. Integrated medicine is better, because it applies the advantages of both.*

Amateur Doctors

Amateur doctors is a term used to refer to those who occasionally provide free services for people they know. I interviewed one of these amateur healers who is 67 years old. According to him, he learned acupuncture and Chinese traditional medicine diagnostic methods from his father. After he graduated from a Chinese-Western medical school, he worked in a Shanghai hospital as an internal doctor. After immigrating to the United States 10 years ago, he gave up his medical practice since he did not need the money.

ENCOUNTERS WITH THE HEALTHCARE SYSTEM

Elderly Chinese are reasonably familiar with the types of problems solved by particular healthcare methods (Guo, 1994). Certain individuals seek Western-style healthcare providers only when they realize that their problems are *Da Mao Bing* (big problems). Likewise, many individuals go to Western-style doctors when they no longer understand the nature of their ailments and when immediate medical attention is needed to release the suffering (Guo, 1994). In these cases, people go to either local Western-style Chinese doctors or hospitals dependent on the status of health insurance coverage.

However, interviews with a large number of elderly Chinese Americans indicated that despite having acknowledged that their problems could be *Da Mao Bing,* many of them did not go to Western-style providers until their problems became too big to handle. Thus there seems to be a space between knowledge of a particular health problem and physical endurance to that problem. When the endurance fades, a healthcare decision is likely to be made. Survey results illustrated the same pattern—a large number of individuals postpone seeing a doctor (Table 9.3).

What are the factors that cause many elderly Chinese hesitation when seeking healthcare? Data gathered from in-depth interviews and surveys suggest that the reality of the American healthcare system and previous encounters with the system may contribute to the process of healthcare-seeking decision making.

Image of the American Healthcare System

As sophisticated as the American healthcare system is, its image is perceived by many elderly Chinese as even more complicated. As one of the key informants in this research described it, the "American healthcare system is like another puzzle that exists in a puzzling like society." Another elderly Chinese complained:

> *There are too many policies and regulations, not to mention doctors and hospitals, even the government agencies have different versions of interpretations on the coverage of Medicaid card. It is just too complicated to know what I can do and what I cannot. That is why so many people will not go to see a doctor if they cannot handle their problem.*

The research highlighted frequently asked questions such as (a) what are Medicaid and Medicare and differences between the two, (b) what the

Table 9.3   Attitude Toward Healthcare Seeking

"For me, to go to see the doctor is my last resort."	
Agree	52 (63%)
Disagree	31 (37%)
Total	83 (100%)

Medicare billing notices mean, (c) why so many doctors do not take the *Lao Ren Card*,[2] (d) what are the differences between private and public hospitals, and (e) how and in what situations one should make a doctor appointment. Consternations about the utilization of public health services are particularly acute for new arrivals to King City, who are often were misinformed and unfamiliar with the American healthcare system. For example, among the 25 structured interview participants, 7 never knew what kind of healthcare benefits they were entitled to, and 6 had not seen a doctor during the previous 2 years of their residency in the United States. All were told by friends that the cost of healthcare in the United States is expensive and one should rather die than be sick.

Earlier immigrants show less concern regarding this issue. Many have either participated in the Medicare program or private insurance programs for many years, and some frequently return to Taiwan and mainland China to receive healthcare.

Hospitals

There are two private hospital facilities located in the central area of King City. Although they are in convenient locations and well known by those in the community, few elderly Chinese have received such services. The majority of elderly Chinese, particularly those who do not have health insurance and who have only Medicaid benefits, travel to the two downtown Manhattan city hospitals, where financial assistance for low-income individuals and a bilingual staff are available, when they need to see a doctor. In the King City area, there are only three doctors willing to treat Medicaid patients.

Because these two hospitals provide special services for low-income individuals of all ethnicity in New York City, they are known in the Chinese American community as the "Poor people hospital" and the "United Nations hospital." During weekdays, these two hospitals' waiting areas are always full of patients. Because of a lack of physicians, a wait of several hours or more is not uncommon, even for people with appointments. "People bring their lunch there, I do too," one elderly Chinese said.

---

[2] *Lao Ren* means old person in Chinese. Since Medicaid and Medicare provide health insurance for eligible elderly people, they are called *Lao Ren Card* in Chinese American communities.

Table 9.4   Frequency of Hospital Visits During the
Past Year

Number of Visits	Total $N = 83$	
0	30	(36%)
1–4	29	(35%)
Over 5	20	(24%)
Missing cases	4	(5%)

Table 9.4 shows the number and frequency of elderly Chinese who utilized hospital services during the year preceding the survey. Although survey results indicate that a large number of elderly Chinese went to hospitals to receive healthcare services at least once in the past year, it is difficult to tell what type of hospital these individuals utilized. Data obtained through interviews with various elderly Chinese reveal that the majority of people who go to these two public hospitals are most likely those who do not have any health insurance coverage or who have only Medicaid. The majority of these individuals are mainland China immigrants, as will be discussed in a later section.

Data obtained through these interviews also indicate that most people only would go to one of these hospitals when they had depleted alternate choices of managing their health problems. The reasons for this resistance are numerous. The inconvenience of traveling, prospect of a long wait; and process of receiving treatment, including the quality of services, appeared to be the major concerns found in the study population.

Problems related to the process of seeking healthcare in Manhattan's downtown hospitals are threefold: scheduling an appointment, completing paperwork, and obtaining appropriate care.

Making an Appointment.   Because of a lack of physicians and an overload of patients, these hospitals require appointments to be made at least two weeks in advance. Moreover, it is not uncommon for patients to wait three or four weeks to see a specialist. Especially for the mainland elderly making an appointment a few weeks ahead is a difficult concept to understand. In mainland China, with the exception being when one wants to see a particular doctor, people normally go to the hospital any time they need to. "It is really a joke, who would know they will be sick four weeks ahead? The only time when I need to see a doctor is because I am ill. Three weeks, by that time it had gotten better by itself," said Mr. Liu, a 64-year-old mainland China immigrant. He spoke with emotion:

I had a fever five months ago. After three days, it was still pretty high. I felt all right, but my wife was worried because my health has not been that good since we came to America. . . . Since I do not have any insurance, I had to go to a hospital. I heard that you have to make an appointment first, but, how, I did not know. By the time I found out from my friend, another two days passed. Finally I called my son and asked him to make an appointment for me . . . my son moved to New Jersey a year ago with his family because he found a new job. Then my son told me I have to wait for three weeks. So, I did not go. I know a friend who knows something about medicine, he came over, and said it was not a big problem. I took some Chinese-made medication, and slept a lot. Two days later, I was all recovered. Later, many people told me, in my situation, I should go to the emergency room, it does not take an appointment. But it is very expensive and you have to wait too.

Paperwork and Tests.   For those who wait and eventually make it to a hospital, there are even more obstacles to overcome. Mr. Yan, a former university professor, shared his story:

A couple of years ago, I caught a flu, and I used some of the Chinese flu drugs I had, but they did not work. So I decided to go to the hospital. After I had waited for almost half a day in the waiting area, an American doctor finally asked me to his office. I know a little bit of English so I told him what was wrong with me. He did not seem to care [for] much of what I said. He asked a nurse over. She brought in a couple [of] forms and asked me to fill them out. It took me twenty minutes to finish them. When he learned that I am 65 years old, he asked to do some examinations and tests from foot to head. I tried to explain to him that I only had a bad flu. But he would not listen to me, and insisted that I must do the test before he can treat me. After several tests, the nurse told me I had to come back some other time to do other tests since their schedule is booked. The whole process of these tests lasted a couple of months. I did not expect so simple a problem caused so complicated [a] process. No wonder America need a healthcare reform.

Mr. Li was diagnosed with a chronic stomach problem 10 years ago when he was still in mainland China. "It was all recovered five years ago before I came here." But he had recently suffered from serious stomach pain for several weeks before relegating himself to bed rest. After one month of self-healing, Mr. Li's stomach did not seem to get better. He decided to take his friend's advice and go to one of the hospitals for professional help.

I was there all day, but the total time I had with [a] doctor was only ten minutes. The rest [of the] time I was busy filling out the forms and doing all kinds of tests which were unrelated to the reason I went there.

After a few visits, one doctor told him he must go to another hospital for a more sophisticated examination, as the necessary equipment was not available at that location.

Two weeks later, Mr. Li went to the second hospital. Staff at that hospital asked him to provide a financial support statement before they could perform the examination. As he was unable to provide the statement, the hospital asked him to return 10 days later for an interview with a social worker to assess the possibility of obtaining Medicaid. Unfortunately, he missed the scheduled appointment because his translator was unavailable. He managed to have someone write a letter for him and address it to the hospital. In the letter Mr. Li requested a new appointment and asked if the hospital could find a bilingual staff person for him. Three weeks later he received a reply from the hospital. They informed him that they set up a new interview for him and that bilingual staff would be available, but that he would have to wait an additional two weeks.

During the two months of waiting, Mr. Li continued self-treatment by using all kinds of Chinese herbal and Chinese-made Western medications. He said he "was all better" by the time he received the final clearance note from the hospital.

The process took a couple of months before I could do that test. If the problem had been really serious, I would be dead before they can start to find out why. Good thing the problem was not that serious, and I did not rely on them.

Quality of Service.   Among the 15 individuals interviewed who had been to these Manhattan hospitals for treatment, only 3 said they had no complaint about the services. Mr. Zhang, a 67-year-old former chief engineer in mainland China, is one of these three informants. When I asked him to speak of his first and last visits to the hospital, he showed a little embarrassment and said he did not have a story to tell. But he had heard other people's experiences and said:

What should we expect from that type of hospital? We all know we go there because we do not have another better choice. We should appreciate at least we have a place to go. This hospital is cheaper, and we want to save money. We made our own choice, so do not complain.

Mr. Zhang's wife has a different attitude:

Yes, it is true that we go there is because it is cheaper, and we do not want to spend hundreds of dollars just for one antibiotic shot. But all hospitals should have one principle regardless of what class of people they serve, that is humanism. I have only been there twice, but what I received from the doctors was a far way from humanism. I do not mind much about waiting. But I cannot stand the way they looked at you, as if you are a worthless person. The doctor I saw was the worst doctor I have seen anywhere. Even the barefoot doctors are better; at least they treated me with sympathy. That doctor did not even bother to look at me much. Two questions and everything was over, before I had a chance to explain anything. That has nothing to do with the type of hospital. The problem is the doctor.

Do not say that. Who wants to work for that type of hospital? No money, and lots of patients. The doctors who are willing to work there are sacrificing their benefits. After all day long with no stop in working hours, who has energy? We should not complain too much, Mr. Zhang added.

Miss Li, a nursing school graduate, rushed from mainland China to King City 2 years ago to take care of her severely ill parents. (Her parents and two sisters immigrated to the United States some 8 years before.) Shortly after her father was diagnosed with Babinski's syndrome 3 years ago, her 72-year-old mother experienced high blood pressure and other symptoms such as weakness and fatigue. The two sisters decided to take their mother to one of the public hospitals, but this idea was rejected by their uncle who had been living in the United States for more than 20 years. "He knows all about the American public hospital situation," Miss Li said. The two sisters insisted, as they were afraid their weakened mother could not tolerate the increased blood pressure. They went to the emergency room one morning and did not leave the hospital until 7 o'clock that night. The next morning, Mother Li lost her speech and could not move. She was taken to the hospital again and diagnosed with cerebral schistosomiasis, "caused by high blood depressor," according to Miss Li.

During the Cultural Revolution my mother had developed high blood pressure. But a doctor found out that the type of blood pressure she has was different than most other people. It was caused by the tensity of the nervous system. So the doctor only prescribed a kind of medication for nervous sedation. She became better after that, especially after the Cultural Revolution and before she came to America she never had high blood pressure again. But her blood pressure went up ever since she came to America. My father's health condition definitely gave a lot of pressure on her. When she was in that hospital, after being sent to various departments for tests, she was completely exhausted when the doctor gave her some high blood pressure depressor. She and both my sisters thought that the doctor must have known everything about Mother since they did all day tests on her. . . . After it happened, my sisters called me (she was still in China), I asked several doctors, they all said it was caused by the depressor. . . . My sisters made a big mistake by taking my mother to that hospital. I went to that hospital many times to see my mother after I came here.

During those three months, I witnessed many things about that hospital, from nursing care skills to the treatment process. I was a nurse, and had worked in a small hospital (in mainland China) for 10 years. Not only [are] the nurse's clinical hands-on skills so bad here, their attitudes are also far worse than in China. Because it is a public hospital, and most patients there are poor, and cannot speak English, they treated them with ice faces. . . . the doctors also try new drugs on their patients. I heard so many people complain about these things. What I want to tell you is this: once you walked into that hospital you would have a problem if you did not have one before you walked in; the problem would be bigger if you only had a small one; and you would die if you had a big one.

Although Miss Li can express only her personal feelings, her general attitude toward public hospitals in New York City was shared by many individuals encountered throughout my field research.

Attitude Toward Western-Style Doctors

As discussed in a preceding section, there are about 200 licensed Western-style Chinese physicians in the area of King City. The majority of elderly Chinese relies on these Western-trained Chinese doctors in King City, especially those elderly persons who have Medicare or private health insurance coverage. Table 9.5 shows that during the past 12 months among 83 elderly Chinese respondents, 33% said they did not visit any Western-style doctors, and 63% said they visited one at least once.

The attitudes of these elderly Chinese toward Western-style doctors were mixed. Some believed that their doctors were very good, and they were happy with them. Others thought their doctors were ordinary and neither better nor worse than other doctors. However, a large number of individuals felt that there were very few good doctors in King City and the

Table 9.5   Frequency of Visiting Western-Trained
Chinese Doctors During the Past Year

Number of Visits	Total $N = 83$
0	27 (33%)
1–4	21 (25%)
Over 5	32 (38%)
Missing cases	3 (4%)

doctors' skills were not as good as they had expected. Table 9.6 illustrates
the general attitude of the surveyed population toward its doctors. Among
83 surveyed individuals, 47% thought there were a few good doctors in
King City, while 22% held the opposite view, and 31% indicated that they
did not know. Also, 56% of the respondents said the doctors they had seen
were not as good as they had expected; only 19% of the respondents dis-
agreed, and the rest remained neutral.

In a discussion with several key informants about the survey results, I
learned that there were several reasons a number of individuals indicated
neutrality in responding to the survey's questions: They simply may have
never visited any doctors, and they may have not wanted to complain.
One key informant, Mr. Fan, said:

*Especially people who are my age, we do not like to complain, com-
plaining is not a very good thing. Have you heard the saying, "elderly*

Table 9.6   Attitude Toward Western-Style Doctors in King City

"There are few good doctors whom we could see in this area."	
Agree	39 (47%)
Disagree	18 (22%)
Don't know	26 (31%)
"The skills of the doctors I have seen here are not as good as I had expected."	
Agree	46 (56%)
Disagree	16 (19%)
Don't know	21 (25%)
"We know our health condition better than doctors do."	
Agree	65 (78%)
Disagree	15 (18%)
Don't know	3 (4%)

$N = 83$

Chinese only complain 20% of what they are suffering"?[3] *But if they think you are not bad, and someone else asked them about you, they will put in many good words for you. Because that is what the Confucians believed. However, if someone asked me about you, and I know you are not that good, I would say to that person I do not know. But if you were a really bad person, then I would say 'he is not that good.' You understand. That is the Chinese way.*

Mongolian and Xiao Er Ke Doctors.   One day while walking into the elevator in the Chinese Senior Center in King City, three elderly Chinese women walked out, and one of them said, "He is another *Mongolian* doctor." That night Mr. Fan asked, "You never heard this term?" He sounded very surprised. According to Mr. Fan, in Mongolia, as well as in other nomadic areas, the few doctors who traveled to see patients were mostly self-taught. They treated not only people but also animals. They knew a bit of everything, but they were not good at anything. Somehow this expression has become a commonly used term by many Chinese Americans in King City to refer to the "ordinary" doctors. "But these doctors in King City are all medical school graduates, how could they be that bad?" I asked. "Xiao Guo, there are many things you need to learn, let me tell you," Mr. Fan said.

It does not literally mean they are lacking in medical knowledge. They probably do know a lot since they all have degrees. But it is the way they treat you. If you are elderly, they know they have to treat you, because otherwise the news is going to spread out in the community, then their faces would not look good. But they really do not want to treat you, because you are old. . . . Why? First is the money. They can not make much money on us. Most people who go to see them have the Lao Ren Card, *so they cannot make much money. Well, if you are a first timer, then they have reasons to do all kinds of test on you, then they can make some money. But if you are [an] old patient, they cannot do that all the time, unless you told him something new, then they can do the tests again. Second, most of us have chronic problems, we go there because these problems are bothering us. They know it is difficult to cure these problems. So every time you call them, they have to make a room for you, then you are not*

---

[3] The first time I heard this saying was at a workshop regarding elderly rights. A Chinese American attorney used the statement to demonstrate how vulnerable elderly Chinese are in American society. I have since learned that elderly Chinese do not usually complain about their problems.

happy because after you have seen them for many years nothing has improved. Especially many elderly want to tell doctor everything, what they ate, how was their sleep . . . because they want the doctor to understand why they are not feeling well. But some doctors do not have the patience to listen, time for them is money. They want to see other patients, not you. So what is happening is that as soon as you walked in, they will just talk to you for a few minutes; then say: "I am giving you a new medication. It is very good." Many elderly will feel hopeful because they are getting new medications. But a lot of people are not happy, we know what they try to do. That is [why] we call these doctors "Mongolian doctor."

What Mr. Fan said is agreed with by many of the elderly Chinese interviewed. In addition to *Mongolian* doctor, another commonly used term, *Xiao Er Ke* refer to the same type of doctors.

The first time I heard this term being used was while accompanying an 87-year-old Chinese woman to her doctor's appointment in King City. Mother Chen came from Taiwan about 14 years ago. She has had diabetes for 7 years, and she has also been suffering from bronchitis, asthma, high blood pressure, and arthritis. In her own words, "I am a useless, and hopeless *Lao Bing Hao* (one who is always ill). No doctor likes to see me around. I cause headaches for them." She is a person with a great sense of humor. "Otherwise I could have been the West Heaven[4] a long time ago," she said in response to a compliment on her positive attitude.

Referring to the appointment afterward, she said, "Ha, they are all the same." Not understanding what she meant by that, I asked again, "Is he (the doctor) good?" "Hi(!), just like Dr. Cai, he is another *Xiao Er Ke* doctor," she said. *"Xiao Er Ke?"* I puzzled for a second. A common Chinese use of this term refers to a kind of miser who will not spend even one penny on others without doing serious thinking.

This term also means the department of Pediatrician.[5] What people like Mother Chen refer to by using this term has two underplayed meanings. First, there are people who think that little children have only little problems, thus being a pediatrician does not mean he or she has a great amount of knowledge. Second, children are easily satisfied if the doctor gives them sweet-tasting medications. Therefore, doctors who seem unwilling to listen to elderly patients, have little idea about their patients' problems and usually rush patients out of their offices, perscribing "new medications."

---

[4] West Heaven is a term dubbed for death in Chinese.

[5] In Chinese, *Xiao* means little or small, *Er* means children, and *Ke* means department.

Good Doctors.   The purpose of the previous discussion is not to make any judgments on the performance of Western-style doctors in King City; it is to demonstrate some of the reasons that have caused the gap between some physicians and their elderly patients. Actually, although doctors were dubbed as *Mongolian* or *Xiao Er Ke* by elderly Chinese, they were thought of, by others, as good doctors. Of interest is the perception of "good doctor." Notably, few individuals actually spoke about a good doctor in reference to his or her medical skills. The majority, however, thought that a good doctor should be a "nice person" and give the medications elderly patients want.

The concept of a nice person was the central theme when elderly Chinese discussed their doctors. In the conversation with Mother Chen, she said the doctor she had just seen was "another *Xiao Er Ke* doctor," like Dr. Cai. She said that Dr. Cai had been a long time family doctor to her and her husband since they immigrated to the United States 14 years ago. "Why are you still seeing him if you think he is a *Xiao Er Ke* doctor?" I asked. "We like him, he is a nice man, kind, honest and patient," Mother Chen replied. Before I had finished, "But doctors are supposed to treat your problems with skills. . . ?" Mother Chen already knew what was asked:

> *It is not easy to find a skilled doctor here. They [are busy] making money with other kinds of people. They only take private insured patients. We have no chance to see them, and they all have big heads . . . So the doctors we can see are all the same in skills. We feel lucky enough to have him.*
>
> *[I saw this doctor today because] I heard from the radio he is good at treating my problems. Although I never believed it, I still thought . . . to try my luck.*
>
> *[He is a* Xiao Er Ke *doctor because] he only asked me a few questions, and gave me the exact same prescription as I have been given by Dr. Cai for five years—another cough syrup.*[6]

Later that day, I checked with Mr. Yang, a key informant, about *Xiao Er Ke* doctors and "nice persons." Mr. Yang said:

> *Although we know the health problems we have are impossible to get rid of, we do want to get some comfort from the doctor that our problems*

---

[6] The term "cough syrup" refers to a kind of medication that would neither help nor hurt a person's condition.

are not getting too deteriorated. We also know all doctors here are pretty much the same, so if a doctor wants [to] talk to you, shares his sympathy, tells you that you will be all right, nothing will become serious, and he can give the prescription we wanted, that is enough. That's all many people wanted.

So what kind of medication do you want from your doctor? I asked.

I know I will bring all the problems I have now to see the god. But just like many others, I do not want to suffer too much before that day arrives. So if the medication can make me feel better, that is enough.

Doctors' Viewpoint

Data obtained from interviews with seven Western-style Chinese physicians generated several perspectives regarding elderly Chinese health and healthcare in King City. Most of these doctors felt that the elderly Chinese in this community are quite resourceful in dealing with their health problems. However, they expressed that the wide range of healthcare resources often causes conflict with treatment procedure.

Lack of a Preventive Concept.   It was surprising to learn that some doctors thought the elderly Chinese lack a preventive concept, since research data accumulated from interviews overwhelmingly demonstrated that the concept of prevention directs the daily activities of many elderly Chinese. According to Dr. Wu, a well known Asian American physician in New York City, the reason she thought elderly Chinese in general lack a preventive concept is that most elderly individuals do not seek healthcare until the problems become serious. "Few of them regularly go to their doctors to have their yearly physical check up, for example," Dr. Wu stated.

It is true that a large number of elderly Chinese does not have its yearly physical. Survey results indicate that only 24.3% of the population reported having an annual physical every year, and 36% of the respondents reported that their last physical examination was done before 1990 (Table 9.7).

Survey results also indicate that among the list of reasons given for missing a yearly checkup, the three major reasons are (a) "knowing one's my own health condition, (b) having too little money, and (c) traveling to doctor is an inconvenience. (Table 9.8).

Doctor Shopping.   The practice of doctor shopping is a major concern frustrating physicians in King City. It appears that many elderly Chinese do not have regular doctors, and thus they frequently go to different doctors.

Table 9.7   Yearly Physical Examinations

Yearly	20	(24%)
Not Yearly	58	(70%)
Missing cases	5	(6%)
Last physical		
Before 1990	30	(36%)
In 1991	7	(9%)
In 1992	16	(19%)
In 1993	22	(27%)
Missing cases	8	(9%)
Total	83	(100%)

Even among those who have a regular physician, it is common for a patient to see two doctors at one time without notifying either of the physicians. Dr. Zhang said:

> *It creates a big headache for me, I never know what kind of medications they have been taking. I know many of them are not satisfied with their doctors because they think that their problems have not gotten better as quickly as they wanted. But to see different doctors at the same time would only make the situation worse. We never know the real history of their problems.*

Dr. Zhang stated that he gets new patients all the time. Although he knows these patients have seen other doctors "they would not tell me what kind of doctors they saw before."

Table 9.8   Reasons for Not Having a Yearly Physical

Reason	Total Response	
I know my health condition.	25	(30%)
It is too expensive.	20	(24%)
It is not convenient to do it.	17	(21%)
I do not know where I can do it.	8	(10%)
There is no difference if I do or not.	6	(7%)
No time to do it.	2	(2%)
Other	2	(2%)
Missing cases	3	(4%)
Total	83	(100%)

One day I was asked by an elderly Chinese to accompany her to a university health clinic. Because there were no Chinese-speaking doctors in the clinic, I served as translator. It was Mother Gao's first visit to this clinic; an American physician asked her to provide her previous doctor's name and address so that a comprehensive analysis of her problem could be undertaken. Mother Gao asked me to check on the possibility of her not having to name her doctor. Later I asked Mother Gao why she did not want to reveal her doctor's identity. She said, "Dr. Cheng is a very nice man. I did not tell him about this. I do not want to hurt his feelings."

Unhealthy Lifestyle.   Dr. Hui is a very popular doctor among elderly Chinese in King City, as he is the only doctor in this community who accepts elderly patients regardless of insurance status. Almost every elderly Chinese knows him, and a large number have been treated by him. The reputation of his medical skills is mixed, but he is generally viewed as a nice person among the elderly population. "He will give you the medications for free if you do not have the money," one informant said. Although he specializes in cardiology and internal medicine, Dr. Hui sees patients with various health problems and even treats his patients with acupuncture.

In discussions regarding common health problems found in the elderly Chinese population in this community, Dr. Hui revealed that high blood pressure, heart disease, arthritis, stomachache and intestinal diseases, followed by diabetes and hepatitis, are among the most prevalent health problems. A major factor, according to Dr. Hui, is that many elderly Chinese lack knowledge regarding how to prevent these health problems. He commented:

> *For example, many people love pork, especially the fatty part. Many people cannot afford to buy other meats than pork, they always like to buy the cheapest parts. They also like to cook the foods with various strong-tasting ingredients. Some of them will cause the high blood pressure if they are frequently consumed.*

According to Dr. Hui, other factors such as a lack of exercise, the pressures of being in an unfamiliar social environment, and problems generated by intergenerational conflicts in many elderly Chinese American families also play an important role in the prevalence of high blood pressure and other health problems.

Financial Factors.   All of the doctors interviewed believed that concern for healthcare costs was an additional reason many elderly Chinese wait to see a doctor. Dr. Wang stated:

I had several patients who complained that they had been coughing for weeks, so I ordered the X-ray test for them. There were also a couple of cases who complained about their body pains and injuries, so I sent them to the hospital to have an X-ray. But they never did it. I believe it is a matter of money, since most of these patients did not have any insurance. There is another factor as well, that is the nature of the problem. For the patients I just mentioned, they probably thought they were not that serious. Yes, the inconvenience is another reason. If they go there, they have to find someone who speaks English, as you probably know, many elderly do not want to ask for [a] favor, especially if it is a difficult one.

Money sometimes plays a big role in this, but it is not the only factor. People from Mainland China, Hong Kong or other areas of Asia might take money as the major factor. But there are people who come from Taiwan who also will not come to see doctors unless they had no other choice.

American patients have a completely different behavior pattern than the Chinese in terms of spending money on doctors. Americans think that money should not be the concern when it comes to the health. They think it is [a] must expense. They would use a credit card if they do not have the cash. Elderly Chinese think of this issue a little differently. They think the money spent on their healthcare is extra, they would rather save it for other purposes. Therefore, I have to say that the Medicare system is really doing a good job on this issue. Most elderly patients who come to see me have Medicare benefits. . . . Without any insurance, nobody would come here unless it was an emergency.

Faith in Western Medicine.   For almost all *Da Mao Bing* (big problems), especially the acute problems, the elderly Chinese were quite convinced of the effectiveness of Western medical treatment. This faith in Western medicine was a generalized one. Even when elderly patients were not satisfied with their doctors' treatment, they would generally blame that particular doctor, but the confidence in Western medicine was still maintained. When this situation occurs, the elderly patient seeks another doctor, resulting in the doctor shopping frequently found in King City.

Even to those who do not have healthcare insurance, to consult with other types of Western-trained doctors, such as a nonlicensed allopathic Chinese doctor, or public hospitals, is the first choice made when starting to experience an acute problem. Some, however, prefer integrated doctors since these individuals also have some training in Western medicine.

Doctors of Chinese Medicine.   As discussed in a preceding section, there are more than 74 practitioners of Chinese medicine in King City. Despite the fact that few of these practitioners can accept any health insurance or Medicare and Medicaid, a considerable number of elderly Chinese frequently utilize their services. Table 9.9, on the following page, shows that

Table 9.9   Frequency of Visiting Chinese
Medicine Doctors During the Past Year

Number of Visits	Total N = 83	
0	49	(59%)
1–4	16	(19%)
Over 5	16	(19%)
Missing cases	2	(3%)

38% of the surveyed population reported seeing Chinese medicine doctors at least once in the previous year. Of the total number surveyed, 19% indicated that they had visited Chinese medicine doctors over five times.

According to interviews with various types of traditional Chinese medicine practitioners, and from personal observation, the health problems elderly Chinese bring to these Chinese medicine doctors are predominantly chronic, including anemia, diabetes, heart disease, and other functional problems. However, there are also considerable numbers of elderly Chinese who seek these practitioners for treatment and explanations for problems that Western medicine doctors fail to treat and diagnose. Interestingly, according to several Chinese medicine doctors, many people come to see them after they are diagnosed by Western medicine doctors. Dr. Zhang said:

> It is not surprising. Many people believe that the diagnosis method of Western medicine is more effective than Chinese medicine's since they have good equipment. But they consider Chinese medicine to have better treatment methods than the Western's. Especially for the elderly people, they are afraid of the side effects of Western medication, and they know Chinese medicine herbal treatment is holistic and effective in the long-term, yet without side effects. That is why they came here for treatment.

In addition to the five healthcare facilities advertising integrated[7] practice, there are many Chinese medicine practitioners in King City, especially those who recently came from mainland China, who provide integrated treatment.[8] Because the integration approach has achieved great success in mainland China, the practice of integrated medicine in

---

[7] The integration of Chinese and Western medicines.
[8] Every Chinese medicine college in mainland China requires students to take Western medicine courses in both theory and practice.

King City has attracted a large number of Chinese Americans, as well as non-Chinese populations. Several of this type of practitioner interviewed indicated that they often had elderly patients request advice regarding which approach should be used to treat their problems, as many practitioners provide free consulting services. Dr. Liu said:

> *Since we all have some knowledge about Western medicine, we would suggest to them to see Western medicine doctors if we believed it was the best way. That is why so many people call us and come in to ask advice, they trust us.*

Some elderly Chinese said explanations they received from Chinese medicine doctors they saw for their health problems made sense and were very convincing. One elderly Chinese man, who immigrated to the United States 20 years ago, stated:

> *The* Zhong Yi *(Chinese medicine doctor) I saw in King City is very different from those I had seen in Chinatown 10 years ago. Over in Chinatown, they all were too traditional. I could not understand their language, although they sounded familiar. That was why I have not visited any Chinese Medicine doctors for 10 years. The one I just saw a couple of weeks ago in King City is very knowledgeable about Western medicine. After I told him about my symptoms and illness history, he knew exactly what kind of Western medications I took, and not only told me the symptom I am having is because of the side effect from the Western drug I have been taking, but also he explained to me why. He is very convincing, and I have learned a lot about Chinese medicine since I saw him.*

According to several Chinese medicine doctors interviewed, a large number of their elderly patients were mainland China immigrants. Dr. Lo remarked:

> *It is because people from the Mainland know more about Chinese medicine, as you know Chinese medicine in mainland China has equal status with Western Medicine. But in Taiwan; it is different. I had quite [a] few elderly patients who came from Taiwan, they questioned a lot, and they always seemed too suspicious about what I said to them. But not the Mainland immigrants. I do not have to explain too much, they know what I mean.*

However, these Chinese medicine practitioners all agreed that the elderly patients do not constitute the bulk of their practice. A major problem is the cost, since none of these doctors can accept any insurance coverage.

CONCLUSION

As previously noted, there are several approaches to the decision-making process in terms of stages and phases, such as Weaver's Model of Spanish Americans in New Mexico (1970), Fabrega's Model of Illness Behavior (1974), and Louie's Model of Chinese Americans in San Francisco (1975). Those approaches that attempt to explain the healthcare decision-making process with a systematic model are found to have value in preliminary assessment of healthcare seeking behaviors and decision making (Pelto & Gove 1992). But the data from King City illustrate a complexity of healthcare behavior and decision making in the elderly Chinese population. The great variety of healthcare possibilities in King City and the eclecticism of healthcare seeking behavior found in the study population suggest that these models relatively are not useful.

The data from King City present a complex picture of healthcare seeking behavior in the elderly Chinese population. The factors which affect elderly Chinese access to modern healthcare facilities are multiple and vary among individuals. Although many individuals have faith in Western medicine and acknowledge that certain problems should be treated by Western-style health providers, they will seek medical assistance only when they can no longer handle their problems. There is also a large number of individuals who engage in a mixed healthcare seeking pattern—doctor shopping, getting advice from integrated practitioners before making a healthcare decision, seeking treatment from a Chinese medicine doctor after obtaining a diagnosis from a Western-style doctor, and seeing additional doctors to get further help. The factors that might have generated such patterns can be summarized in the following points:

1. Especially among the new arrivals, who are often misinformed and misled by characterizations about the American healthcare system, fear must often be generated before people pursue needed healthcare services. At the same time, the complexity and problems within the American healthcare system itself certainly enhance such fears.

2. Many individuals experience various difficulties in the process of seeking healthcare. The requirement of making an appointment several weeks in advance and long waits in hospitals discourage elderly

Chinese, especially those who do not have healthcare insurance, from seeking healthcare services.

3. A substantial amount of paperwork and complicated tests by machines used in the process of modern healthcare create a biased attitude toward Western healthcare facilities among many elderly Chinese. Many individuals think that Western medicine doctors in this community are less skilled than doctors in China because they rely too much on machine-based diagnosis rather than their clinical experiences.

4. Data also show that certain groups of people believe that Chinese herbal medicines and Chinese-made Western medications are better than American-made medications for treatment of their health problems, and the one purpose of visiting a doctor is to obtain medications. Even for those who believe in Western medications, the alternative resources available to them make it unnecessary to see doctors.

5. The various types of Chinese medicine practitioners, especially those who practice integrated medicine, provide an important alternative healthcare method for those dissatisfied with Western medicine, and who maintained a strong faith in Chinese medicine. Despite the fact that none of the Chinese medicine practitioners in King City can accept any health insurance, a large number of elderly Chinese, especially those from mainland China, still frequently utilize the services provided by these practitioners. It is interesting to note that many people seek Chinese medicine doctors for treatment after obtaining a diagnosis from a Western-style physician.

6. Language barriers, high costs of healthcare, and expectation conflicts also all contribute to healthcare decision making.

The elderly Chinese of King City provide an example of the complex patterns of change and experimentation that occur when people with a very rich culture of health beliefs and practices move into an economic and cultural environment dominated by the technologically advanced American healthcare system. This confrontation between the people and the healthcare system of King City highlights the differences between the two healthcare systems; it also exposes many of the difficult and cumbersome features of the American healthcare system.

The elements of this confrontation can be conceptualized at two levels: macro and micro.

Macro-Level

To many elderly Chinese, the American healthcare system presents a formidable image. The countless regulations, high costs of care, and divergent policies in different healthcare facilities often generate a great fear of accessing healthcare services. In rationalizing their fears about the American healthcare system, many individuals attribute it to the sharp difference of the two cultures in values, norms, and social systems. As an informant put it, the "American healthcare system is like another puzzle-that exists in a puzzling-like society."

Micro-Level

This level includes the problems and difficulties that elderly Chinese experience in the process of healthcare seeking.

The American healthcare system, particularly that portion used for serious illness, is made more inaccessible because of the economic costs as well as the social complexity. Visits to healthcare facilities are complicated social encounters, with large amounts of paperwork, complex instructions to follow, elaborate testing procedures, and other hurdles. In contrast to the Chinese traditional and nontraditional health beliefs and practices, the American system, with its technological and regulatory complexity, has many obscure and relatively inaccessible features. The presence of complex equipment, even in the average doctor's office; elaborate clinics and hospitals; and complicated treatments present major obstacles to understanding, portability, and access.

The hardships that elderly Chinese encounter in dealing with healthcare providers further confirm their presumptions and stereotypes about the American healthcare system. As a result, in addition to that social and economic complexity placed behind a screen of language differences, accessing the healthcare system is truly a formidable undertaking. At every turn the elderly Chinese, even those quite seriously ill, are strongly discouraged from getting needed services.

REFERENCES

Carp, F. M., & Kataoka, E. (1976). Health care problems of the elderly of San Francisco's Chinatown. *The Gerontologist, 16*(1), 30–38.

Chen, P. N. (1979). A study of Chinese-American elderly residing in hotel rooms. *Social Casework, 60*(2), 89–95.

Chen, V. Wen Chee (1989). Communication and conflict between American born Chinese and their immigrant parents. *Dissertation Abstracts International, 49*(12), 3883A.

Cheng, E. (1978). *The elder Chinese.* San Diego State University, Center on Aging.

Cheung, M. (1989, September). Elderly Chinese living in the United States: Assimilation or adjustment? *Social Work,* 457–461.

Chinese Business Directory. (1994). *World Journal Press.* New York: Whitestone.

Fujii, S. M. (1976). Elderly Asian Americans and use of public services. *Social Casework, 57*(3), 202–207.

Guo, Z. (1994). *Health, medicine, and beliefs—Chinese American elderly in a developing urban community.* Unpublished doctoral dissertation, University of Connecticut, Storrs.

Hessler, R. M. (1975). Intraethnic diversity: Health care of the Chinese Americans. *Human Organization, 34*(3), 253–262.

Ikels, C. (1983). *Aging and adaptation: Chinese in Hong Kong and the United States.* Hamden, CT: Archor Books.

Kao, Chingyi (1981). *Alternative health care practitioners in a Chinese American community: A preliminary report of findings.* U.S. Department of Education, National Institute of Education, ERIC.

Kleinman, A. (1980). *Patients and healers in the context of culture.* Berkeley: University of California Press.

Liu, W. (1986). Health services for Asian elderly. *Research on Aging, 8*(1), 156–175.

Lum, D., & Cheung, L. Y. S. (1980). The psychological needs of the Chinese elderly. *Social Casework, 61*(2), 100–106.

Nagasawa, R. (1980). *The elderly Chinese: A forgotten minority.* Chicago: Pacific Asian American Mental Health Research Center.

Pelto, G., & Gove, S. (1992). *Developing a focused ethnographic study for the WHO acute respiratory infection control program.* Geneva: WHO/ARI.

Wong, B. (1982). *Chinatown: Economic adaption and ethnic identity of the Chinese.* New York: Holt, Rinehart and Winston.

Wong, E. F. (1980). Learned helplessness: The need for self-determination among the Chinese American elderly. *Journal of Ethnic Studies, 8*(2), 45–62.

Wu, F. Y. T. (1975, June). Mandarin-speaking aged Chinese in the Los Angeles area. *The Gerontologist,* 271–275.

Wysocki, B. (1991, January 15). Influx of Asians brings prosperity to Flushing: A place for new comers. *The Wall Street Journal,* A1.

Ying, Y. W. (1988). Depressive symptomatology among Chinese-Americans as measured by the CES-D. *Journal of Clinical Psychology, 44*(4), 739–749.

CHAPTER TEN

The Changes and Strategies Adopted by the Public Health Services and Medical Society in Japan

Michiyo Mizuno, PHN, MSN, RN

*J*apan is the first Asian country that has successfully adopted and put into practice the medical technologies previously developed in Europe and the United States. Many of the lethal diseases that had raged for centuries, such as tuberculosis and smallpox, were eradicated or nearly conquered by the advanced public health and medical care in Japan. While the medical and health professions in Japan still strive to control the so-called intractable diseases, changes are currently taking place throughout Japanese society, as it evolves ever more rapidly, pose new challenges to those involved in medical care and public health. Some of these challenges are shared by the United States and other developed countries while some are entirely unique to Japan. A rapid increase in the elderly population is one concern that many developed countries now face and will continue to face in the near and far future. Combined with a social security system unique to Japan, however, the issue of a rapidly aging society takes on a different picture, requiring that the government take urgent action simply to cope. In another context, one notes the concepts of health and illness as changing perhaps too slowly in Japan, as advancements in medical science continue to ease harsh suffering from serious diseases.

In this chapter, I describe some of the changes taking place within the context of public health services and medical societies in Japan. More specifically, I discuss how the current healthcare delivery system is being tailored to adapt to a changing society and what new strategies have evolved to face emerging challenges. In explaining the difficulties that society faces in pursuing the new approaches, I will also examine those Japanese cultural characteristics closely related to the delivery of healthcare. Finally, I offer a perspective on the medical and healthcare services in Japan as they relate to the research and analysis detailed in the preceding sections.

Unless stated otherwise, I have taken all data or statistics used in this chapter from the *Vital Statistics of Japan* (1996a) published by the Director-General, Statistics and Information Department at the Minister's Secretariat, Ministry of Health and Welfare. Vital statistics are those obtained from surveys conducted every month in Japan on matters related to births, deaths, fetal deaths, marriages, and divorces.

CHANGES IN DEMOGRAPHY AND FINANCIAL SITUATION

Accelerated Increase of an Aging Population

The population of Japan reached 125,034,000 people. As estimated by the Administration and Management Agency's Statistics Bureau, in 1994. During the post-World War II period, of course, Japanese economy, science, and technology developed rapidly, with dramatic and far reaching effects, including a general alteration in life style, industrial structure, and demographic composition similar to those of Western nations. With progressively expanded productive capacities brought by intensive industrialization, the population has concentrated in urban areas to service and consumes major industrial goods. For this discussion, it is important to note, however, that this segment of the population drawn into urban areas was composed mainly of younger people. Thus the traditional form of the family unit—the eldest son, his wife, and their children living with his old parents to carry on family traditions—began to crumble. Around this time, perhaps by 1965, the expression "a nuclear family" came into existence to describe the new situation. Although the percentage of young couples living with parents 65 years or older is still fairly high in Japan in comparison to Western nations, it did decline from 68% to 55.3% between 1975 and 1994, leaving approximately 40% of the Japanese elderly to live alone or to live only with their respective spouses. It is a trend more eminent in urban communities than elsewhere (Statistics and Information Department at Minister's Secretariat, Ministry of Health and Welfare, 1996b).

On the other hand, advances in medical science improved living standards, and related changes made it possible to rapidly ameliorate the circumstances that surround death in Japan. By 1995, the life expectancy at birth in Japan stood at 76.36 years for males and 82.84 years for females. The dramatic increase in life expectancy at birth and low overall birth rates have exaggerated the aging of the society. Currently, among the leading nations of the world, Japan ranks first in terms of life expectancy at birth and lays claim to a low mortality.

As a result, Japanese society is aging at a faster rate than the other industrialized nations of the world. When the total population is divided into three age groups, the group of under 1 to 14 year olds declined from 35.4% in 1950 to 16.0% in 1995, while the productive group, composed of those between 15 and 64 years and the elderly (65 years and older) rose annually. In particular, the increase in the size of the oldest segment has been significant. According to the 1992 population projections for Japan by the Ministry of Health and Welfare, 21.3% of the total population will be 65 years or older by 2010, again the highest among the industrialized countries of the world.

In Japan, as in Western nations, the birth rate began to drop sharply early in the 1970s and, by 1994, reached an all-time low of 1.46. An upturn in the age at marriage, higher maternal age, and a drop in the number of couples who marry are the current main causes for fewer births in Japan. A trend toward fewer children reflects the changing role of women in society. Japanese women are assuming more important positions in a society that was once a bastion of male dominance, with more women gainfully employed as well. Having fewer children allows more women to consider careers that their parents or grandparents might not have been able to consider. A drop in the birth rate and the resulting shorter child care period also affords more opportunities for women to seek employment outside the home.

As the trend toward fewer births continues, the population will continue to age. In particular, there is a notable increase in the number of elderly who have reached advanced age. In Japan, the percentage of the population 80 years and older to the total mortality accounted for 41.4% in 1994. Finally, in step with the current pace of aging of the population, the number of deaths will begin to rise.

Although mortality itself remained at a level of 700,000 for an extended period across the age spectrum, it reached 820,000 in 1990; and according to population projections for Japan by the Ministry of Health and Welfare (1992), it is expected to reach one million in 1999. After the year 2010, this number will surpass what modern medical care systems have ever had to face.

Precisely, Japan is faced with the problem of a rising mortality, which in turn means an accelerated demand for medical or long-term care for the very old. Among 16,900,000 Japanese elderly age 65 and older in 1995, 1,050,000 were institutionalized while 840,000 remained at home receiving some form of long-term care (Statistics and Information Department at Minister's Secretariat, Ministry of Health and Welfare, 1997). An increasing number of elderly Japanese are receiving long-term care at home. However, in cities in particular, a typical modern Japanese family is composed of only a few members and the ability to care for their own family members is limited. As for the long-term care, the capacity of the individual family is readily exhausted.

Social Security System

Health is related to life. Many problems related to life—poverty, unemployment, illness, injury, and aging—are liable to develop in every segment of society. As we encounter such problems throughout the life span, we cope with them, as we can, to live a healthy life with full responsibility for our actions. In this regard, the governmentally constituted social security system, via Article II X V of the constitution of Japan, was established to guarantee each Japanese a minimum standard for the provision of a healthy and civilized life in modern society.

In fact, the social security system was designed to provide for life and health related problems such as poverty, unemployment, illness, injury, or old age. The Secretariat of the Social Security System Council of the Prime Minister's Office has formally defined the scope of social security as relief provided from public funds for social insurance, social welfare, public health or medical care, and healthcare for the aged (Furuich, 1995).

Certainly public health or medical care is most closely related to our health. The Ministry of Health and Welfare administers, as a central organization, healthcare for community residents and medical care for the sick. However, with bureaucracy come other problems associated with the segregation of departments dedicated to singular functions that may or may not speak to the multiform character of the health issue of concern. On the other hand, local self-governing bodies and public health centers manage community health and provide finely tuned health services to meet the diverse needs of community residents. Particularly, the public health center is an institution established by local governments to carry out preventive measures and administrative work within its jurisdiction. In 1995, there were 847 public health centers across the nation (Nakahara & Shobayashi, 1995).

Medical institutions, which include hospitals, clinics, and maternity clinics, most often belong to the private sector. According to a survey of medical care institutions/hospitals as prepared by the Ministry of Health and Welfare (1996c), private hospitals accounted for 81.8% of the total number of hospitals and 69.6% of the total number of beds in 1994. For their part, national and public hospitals, which in particular purport to promote national policy-based medical care, also include clinical research, education, and training activities.

When a Japanese citizen recognizes a need for medical care, he or she chooses a hospital or clinic to visit and purchases there all medical services needed and as medical services are dispensed under the social insurance system. In other words, patients pay fees for medical services through the public medical insurance system, which is a form of social insurance against injury and illness. As in the United States, for instance, the specific details of those services are decided according to a medical fee schedule. Service prices are set by the government, and the criteria of diseases to be treated and services to be offered are stipulated in detail. Each procedure is categorized with a standard fee prescribed throughout the country regardless of the type of medical institution, where the service is offered, or the category of the health professional who delivers the care.

Rapid Rise in Health Expenditures

Universal medical care and a public pension for all citizens comprise the goals of the Japanese social insurance system. Unlike the United States, however, in Japan all citizens are covered by the medical insurance system. First expanded in step with the country's rapid economic growth, by 1961 the medical insurance system achieved its present universal reach. Taking advantage of this expansion, a greater number of citizens began to utilize medical services and in response to this increasing demand, medical institutions grew rapidly in number with a parallel rise in medical expenses generally. In the ensuing 31 years since the establishment of universal medical insurance (1961 to 1992), national health expenditures, including all medical expenses estimated through the medical insurance and publicly funded medical care systems increased by 46 times (Ministry of Health and Welfare, 1996d).

Health costs are funded by the individual (patient's co-payment at the time of examination), insurance premiums, and public funding. Currently, patients' co-payments amount to nearly 12% of the entire expense. Since 1991, however, health expenditures grew at a rate that exceeded the growth in national income that was marred by sluggish economic growth. If the current slow economic growth affects the base of the national economy and continues into the future, health expenditures will exceed the cost level that the general public can bear.

In terms of the aged and the rapid population rise, cost of care to the aged has surpassed the increase in the total cost of medical care for the nation itself. Even if the Japanese economy recovers in the near future, the health insurance system will not be adequate to deal with this mounting problem of rising medical costs unless radical reform to the current system is made. In 1997, it is clear to see that the Japanese health insurance sytem with coverage for the entire nation as its prerequisite has come to a turning point.

PERCEIVED CHANGES IN THE PATTERNS OF DISEASE AND HEALTH

Medical Triumph over Fatal Diseases

The so-called "adulthood related diseases"—cancers, heart and cerebrovascular diseases—comprise the three primary causes of death in Japan. The mortality from these three clinical entities amounted to 59.7% of the total deaths in 1994. Circumstantially checked, the trend in adulthood related diseases as causes of death, remained between 61% and 62% for a decade after 1979, then began to show signs of a gradual decline. A factor in the background of this change is an increase in mortality for particular types of disease: the population at 75 years and older now survive cerebrovascular and other serious diseases through successful medical treatment while remaining in fragile health, enough to succumb to secondary complications such as pneumonia and bronchitis.

Life expectancy at birth in Japan, which ranks as the highest in the world, is explained by the advancement in medical care and improved lifestyle, which also contribute to the prevention of deaths from adulthood related diseases. In fact, mortality in cerebrovascular diseases specifically, which once surpassed all others in Japan, began to decline after hitting a peak in 1970 and has remained ranked third since 1985. Although cancers have remained the primary cause of death since 1981, and its rise is significant, the age-adjusted mortalities—assuming that the population structure remains the same when mortality is calculated—have almost stabilized among males and declined among females. These trends are explained by the decrease in mortality from gastric cancer in males and cervical cancer in females: the two clinical entities that have been the primary and secondary causes of death among Japanese cancer patients generally. Concerted efforts at mass screenings for cancer, such as those affecting the stomach and cervix, enabled early detection and treatment to ward off the development of possible secondary cancers. Similarly, as a consequence of the progress in medical care, the age-adjusted mortality from heart diseases has been on the decline, although it surpassed that from cerebrovascular diseases in 1985 to rank second and has been on the rise ever since.

Nevertheless, population aging is advancing at a pace greater than the growth of medical or healthcare can match. The 1995 patient survey that purported to gather information on the number of patients who use medical facilities and other pertinent data, such as the situation regarding provision for medical care, as conducted by the Statistics and Information Department, Ministry of Health and Welfare, showed the percentages of in- and outpatients aged 65 and over to have been on the upswing. The rise in the proportion of older inpatients is particularly significant for diseases of the circulatory system, including heart, cerebrovascular, and hypertensive diseases. (Among these, the percentage for cerebrovascular disease is particularly high.) The same pattern prevails among outpatients.

When examining the composition of mortality among Japanese elderly, four distinct characteristics surface:

1. High total mortality,
2. Rise in the percentage of diseases involving the circulatory system,
3. Decline in the percentage of cancers, and
4. Rise in the number of infections such as pneumonia and bronchitis (Orimo, 1992).

Diseases affecting the circulatory system are particularly significant. According to the statistics prepared by a patient survey from the Ministry of Health and Welfare (1995a), the average length of stay at hospitals for patients with diseases of the circulatory system was 74.6 days in 1993, which was second only to 333.3 days for mental disorders. The average total length of stay in hospitals for all diseases measured was 41.9 days. When the figures for mental disorders and tuberculosis are excluded, the average length of stay for the general population was computed at 33.9 days. Of course, there was a tendency for the average length of stay to increase with advanced age: 70.8 days for patients age 65 and over.

It is important here to examine the characteristics of diseases of the circulatory system that afflict the elderly Japanese. Generally, many who suffer from heart or cerebrovascular diseases are also affected by a generalized arteriosclerotic process. As many Japanese adopt a diet similar to that common in Western societies, high in calories and rich in dietary fats, the incidence of arteriosclerotic diseases will rise. According to epidemiological studies, however, the frequency and advances in the stage of arteriosclerosis have not been proven to be as fatal in Japan as in the Western world (Orimo, 1992).

Originally, the Japanese were considered liable to develop hypertensive diseases due to a diet high in salt content. Although vigorous efforts have been made in health education to improve the traditional diet and hypertension medication is available, the hypertensive state still remains a grave risk factor in the development of heart and cerebrovascular diseases in Japan.

Cerebrovascular diseases remain a serious issue in Japan not only because they often prove fatal to the elderly but also because they often leave them in a demented or bedridden state for the remainder of their lives. According to a comprehensive survey on the Living Conditions of People in Health and Welfare, including statistics on households and household members throughout the country, as compiled by the Ministry of Health and Welfare of Japan (1997), 31.7% of the elderly who are currently confined to bed have suffered from an apoplectic stroke. A survey on the incidence and mortality from apoplectic strokes at a city in Japan for a period of five years indicated that the morbidity of stroke was twice the mortality of the illness (Shibata, 1990). As to the cause of dementia in Japan, its incidence due to cerebrovascular diseases is twice that in the United States, and it distinctly outnumbers the incidence of Alzheimer's disease.

As previously stated, the age-adjusted mortalities of adulthood related diseases have slowly decreased due to advancements in medical care, an improved lifestyle, and other factors related to modern social values. Meanwhile the number of deaths continues to rise due to the aging of society on the whole. At the same time, the incidence of adulthood related diseases is rising instead of decreasing. From these figures we may conclude that Japanese have learned to live long while many suffer from chronic diseases.

Japanese Concept of Health

According to the comprehensive survey of the Living Conditions of People on Health and Welfare (Ministry of Health and Welfare, 1997), the percentage of people with medical complaints—those not currently hospitalized but with subjective symptoms of some illness or injury—increases every year, numbering 283.3 per thousand population in 1995. The main subjective symptoms include lumbago, stiffness of the shoulders, and arthralgia of the limbs. The incidence is proportional to age. In 1995, approximately one-half of the people 65 years and over suffered from some medical complaint. Moreover, their age was directly reflected in the frequency at which they visited a medical facility and the duration of treatment. In fact, the percentage of the elderly Japanese to the total number of patients suffering from adulthood related diseases is increasing. Nevertheless, in the aforementioned survey, almost 90% of Japanese considered themselves healthy or healthier than the "average person."

Why is this? Why do Japanese think they are healthy although they may have some physical discomfort? The Ministry of Health and Welfare, aided by a private corporation, investigated people's opinions on issues such as health, medical services, and other related matters in 1995. Interviews specially designed for this purpose were targeted to 2000 men and women 20 years and older (excluding those hospitalized at the time when the survey was conducted) selected from the general public (Ministry of Health and Welfare of Japan, 1996). One-third of all respondents replied that to be healthy means "when one suffers from no illness at all," while this view was voiced by 60.3% of the male respondents who were in their 20s. Among the general respondents, 45% believed that one is healthy "when one does not have an illness that requires medical attention." Moreover, 21% considered that a person is healthy "when he is capable of engaging in daily work and other activities without particular difficulty even if that person regularly sees a physician due to a chronic illness." The proportion of those with the latter view increases with age: 28.1% among those 65 through 74 years and 37.2% among those 75 years and older. The same view was expressed by only 14.1% of those in their 20s. It appears that Japanese tend to base their concept of wellness on their ability to control their lives, rather than their illness, as they age and begin to experience physical frailties.

In the same survey, when asked to choose two important activities for health, respondents rated highly (67.6% and 50.1%, respectively) "making an effort to control one's habits and life-style" (self-management) and "actively doing what is considered to be beneficial for health" (self-help efforts for active health promotion). When classified by age, a similar tendency was observed, but the older group (60 years and over) placed greater emphasis on "managing" personal health, with rating scores of 73.6% for this age group as against approximately 65% for other age groups.

Judging from these results as well as those from other public opinion surveys, Japanese citizens show an active interest in health related matters and energetically pursue health promoting activities. However, the mounting concern for their own health may cause an increase in the percentage of people with medical complaints. In Japan as well, there are many patients who wish to obtain detailed explanations concerning their illness but would not dare to pose questions to their physicians or other medical staff beyond such explanations. In the section reserved for opinions on health or medical services in the survey cited, the wish expressed by the majority of respondents toward medical institution staff was "to give an explanation of their illness, treatment methods, and other pertinent matters to the patient's satisfaction," which far outnumbered the wish for "accurate diagnosis of illness and complete cure." Of all respondents, 49.9% expressed the former. Concerning attitudes upon receiving an explanation by a physician and other medical staff on their illness, on the other hand, the most popular response was: "I want to hear a detailed explanation of my condition, but I actually do not ask" (48.4%). Except those in their 20s, this attitude was expressed more commonly by younger groups. The counterpart to this attitude—"I want to get a detailed explanation of my condition and I ask"—was expressed by only 27.3% of respondents.

Regardless, whether they request an explanation for their illnesses or not, it is undeniable that many Japanese wish to have a more detailed explanation from the medical staff. This may be explained by the current situation, where the incidence of chronic diseases is rising and the need for terminal care urge people to take notice of the patient's decision-making process.

MEASURES TAKEN TO COUNTERACT EMERGING CHANGES

Government Policy Focusing on Home Care

As Japanese industry and populations converge onto the urban scene and the trend toward the greying of society with fewer children advances, disproportion among districts becomes more evident and the needs of people more disparate. Such changes require responsive revisions to the administrative systems related to health services, medical care, and welfare.

One notable change implemented recently in this regard concerns the decentralization of the structure of the national government itself with a corresponding reorganization of previously independent healthcare, medical care, and welfare services. Local governments were granted the power to formulate their own policies to cope with problems associated with an aging society, for example, and to provide their citizens with comprehensive health services. The statute providing for health service for the aged— to implement comprehensive healthcare projects, such as community disease prevention, therapy, and rehabilitation programs—became effective in 1982. The intent of this law was and is to combine steps to prevent adulthood related diseases (i.e., chronic, degenerative conditions, often stemming from an individual's personal lifestyle) with those designed to deal with problems related to the elderly and to delegate to local governments the authority to execute specific functions.

Municipalities, the administrative bodies closest to local residents, both physically and psychologically can provide services tailored and individualized to the expressed needs of the elderly. As a result, in 1990, eight laws concerning welfare (e.g., Amendment to the Welfare Law for the Elderly, ect.) were revised to permit municipal governments to develop a system to provide health and welfare services within a comprehensive design. This amendment was amended several times in the ensuing years.

Such laws stipulate that municipalities will assume responsibility for health and welfare services in an integrated manner, not only for the elderly, but also in matters related to maternal and child health, so as to provide health services throughout all life stages. Thus it became necessary to overhaul and update drastically the framework of community health plans that had been created immediately after the end of the war. The Health Center Law that had been the blanket statute to regulate community public health services was replaced by the Community Health Law, as implemented in April 1997. This law allows the national government, prefectural governments, and municipal governments to share appropriate roles to step up decentralization of authority and meet residents' diversified needs.

Another revision in healthcare policies, made to alleviate the skyrocketing medical costs generally, was designed to reinforce and improve home healthcare services. Medical facilities that admit large numbers of elderly Japanese face ever-rising healthcare costs. Moreover, judging not only from a cost benefit analysis but also from the well-being of the recipients themselves, it is overwhelmingly more advantageous to provide long-term care at home in so far as it is practical to do so. The Japanese elderly, like their counterparts in other countries, prefer to remain at home or in a place where they have lived for some time to the very end if at all possible.

As previously mentioned, however, current lifestyle patterns and family structure do not readily permit successful coping with the problems of long-term care for the elderly Japanese. Families must receive support from others and take advantage of a variety of available services. To meet these needs, resources were utilized in revising the Health Service for the Aged Law in 1991, and the visiting nurse system for the bedridden elderly began operation in selected areas throughout Japan in 1992. Under this system, home nursing care is now reimbursable under the health insurance plan. The government plans to open 5,000 stations for this purpose by the year 2000, but implementation of the intended services will be required for actual provision of resources. By 2000, the community welfare service may constitute a fundamental element of elder care. It will not only fortify the medical insurance system that covers the risk of contracting a disease or developing disability but also serve as a social welfare system for long-term care and general welfare.

The national government had attempted to augment the pension and medical insurance systems ahead of welfare services, such as long-term care. The resulting benefit ratio of pension, medical service, and others, in terms of general social security expenditures, came to 5:4:1. Recognizing clear inadequacies here in terms, "others" (welfare services and public assistance), the Ministry of Health and Welfare advocated reconstructing the social security system to attach more weight to welfare and revise the benefit ratio to 5:3:2 for the twenty-first century (Furuich, 1995).

The issue of home healthcare is not a matter that concerns the elderly Japanese alone. The number of patients who suffer from chronic, terminal, or intractable diseases has also been increasing; these patients require residential medical care services to improve the quality of their lives while staying at home.

In step with these rising needs, the national medical administration prepared legislation for in-home medical care and supported it by formulating a system. As such, the Health Insurance Law was revised in 1994 to define clearly that "management of medical care and nursing care for patients living at home" (i.e., home medical care and visiting nurse services) be covered by medical insurance. The new bill allows patients to administer particular inpatient-type medical care by themselves at home under a physician's guidance, with terminal patients or the bedridden elderly patients to receive pain relief, psychological support, or personal care while staying at a place that is familiar to them. Certainly, advancements in medical technology have made it more possible for such needs to be met. In contrast, the hospital system for care for terminal or bedridden elderly patients is not yet as well regulated.

Health Professionals' Support for Self-Management

In Japan today, the public health standard is considered to be fairly high in relation to the rising awareness of the significance of issues related to public health and socioeconomic status. The public health administration, with health centers at its core, has developed health and medical care services by providing preventive healthcare based on considerations of the well-being of society as a whole. At the same time, although the average length of hospital stays in Japan is longer than in the United States, there is a growing tendency to curtail length of stay via government policies to have the bedridden elderly or demented patients cared for at the community level.

Once preventive medicine and treatment achieve a substantially high level, matters such as preventing the exacerbation of disease, promoting social rehabilitation, and assistance in nurturing an individual's self-care ability will surface as necessary steps to improve the health condition of citizens in general. People must maintain their daily life activities as much as possible even when they suffer from diseases or disabilities. In other words, self-management or self-help efforts are essential, not only as part of primary prevention activities for the healthy and secondary prevention for those with compromised health, but also in a tertiary prevention program for those suffering from a disease or disability. We must strive to prevent diseases so that all people may enjoy quality of life within the scope of their limitations.

Health professionals should provide services to recipients in an individualized manner at an appropriate location. Remaining in an environment that the recipient is familiar with, he or she is more likely to exercise self-management and assume responsibility for self-care. It is important that individuals are motivated to make choices for treatment and self-manage insurance for health, medical, and welfare services. Health professionals must be able to educate their patients to recognize and understand their health status or the nature of their illness and be able to cope with associated problems as they arise.

If a patient is to participate in self-care, exchange of information and trust between patient and professional are essential. The concept of patient self-care has found wide acceptance among nurses (Ashworth, 1992). In particular, patient satisfaction is gained by allowing him or her to assume personal responsibility for medical care or treatment through working with physicians and other health professionals. Certainly, the obligation to disclose information regarding an illness and other relevant matters to patients also requires clarity and compassion.

In terms of community healthcare, it is important that the medical institution function as a member of the community where it resides, taking positive steps to provide information and deliver consistent quality medical care within the context of community relations. Although commercialization of medical care is rejected and advertising by medical institutions is banned by the Medical Service Law in Japan, specifically because of the special nature of the services, patients and their families still need appropriate information related to medical institutions in order to select a suitable facility. While considering the public nature of medical services, health professionals should strive to give such information to as many patients as possible.

Undoubtedly, the types of available services and service providers are increasing. With the greater availability of more diversified services, there is a corresponding need for them to be offered to the public in a comprehensive manner. Improvements in the quality and quantity of services and service providers also require a coordinated system to aid the Japanese in making the most of their choices.

CULTURAL IMPLICATION OF HEALTHCARE ISSUES

Japan is an Asian country that retains its unique cultural heritage, and upon which its present healthcare system has been built. Chao (1992) referred to healthcare as an expression of human caring and stated that the healthcare system included peoples' beliefs and patterns of behavior as governed by cultural rules. When we provide healthcare services, it is important that we pay due regard to patients' cultural implications. Thus, it is important to describe how Japanese healthcare needs are related to cultural rules on health related behavior.

Relationship Between Patients and Physicians in Japan

As described earlier, patient self-care allows them to confront their disease while still taking advantage of the quality of life available to them. Availability of information is an indispensable part in this process. Because contemporary medicine is focused mainly on highly specialized treatment, related information has not been available to patients and their families in a form they can readily understand. Moreover, physicians often assume a traditional paternalistic posture and act on the belief that they practice their art *for* the benefit of their patients. In such a setting, they rarely provide the kind of information that patient and family need.

Traditionally, the physician-patient relationship is formed as authoritarian in nature. The patient accepts the instructions given by the physician passively and is not expected to do more. When interfacing with a physician, many Japanese patients remain passive even when they desire to learn more about their own physical condition. In fact, they tend to leave the entire matter related to their medical care to the physician, even when it is important for them to participate actively in their own care.

Faced with the trauma of disease or injury, Japanese patients will often relegate their bodies to the doctor's care. They also try to cope with attending psychological difficulties in the same way, by avoiding them and then entrusting them to the care of other people. Okaya (1988), for example, in a piece of qualitative research on the coping style of 25 Japanese cancer patients who had undergone operations, found 6 distinct coping patterns. When patients underwent an operation, they left their own bodies "to the physician's care." Only one-half of former patients resorted to a style of "seeking information."

Once Japanese relegate their bodies to physicians, they are likely to obey them (even blindly) to maintain a cordial relationship. As a form of coping often favored by Japanese, it does not necessarily mean a renunciation of the coping itself. Unlike Western patients, the confidence Japanese place in their physicians is not necessarily based on the principle of a conventional relationship. Many Japanese feel at ease when they relegate their bodies to physicians, or place extreme confidence in them. That they do this "blindly" enables them to continue and to support their obedience to their physician.

The provision of medical services based on an adequate explanation given to the patient has familiar roots in U.S. and European cultures. The Japanese are not altogether ready to communicate openly with physicians, request an adequate explanation, or arrive at some form of agreement. Unlike Western patients, Japanese are culturally inhibited from expressing their feelings openly. Japanese often *hope* that the person they are communicating with will understand their true intent beyond what words are used. Such is the cultural style that shapes human relationships in Japan.

Japanese often try to judge a situation through interactions with others. For example, according to a survey on cancer patients' knowledge of the true nature of their illness learned from family members who cared for them during the terminal stage, about 20% of family members stated that "the patient was notified and knew the nature of his illness"; 43.8% said that "the patient sensed the nature of his illness"; and 28.8% said "the patient was neither notified nor sensed." This study, part of the socioeconomic survey of vital statistics by the Ministry of Health and Welfare (1996e) contained 2,810 responses collected in 1994 in 11 prefectures in Japan. As a rule, the diagnosis of cancer is disclosed to only a limited number of patients in this country. Many cancer patients probably sense the nature of their illness because of their physical condition and others' reactions to them. As the survey shows, then, there are a number of patients and family members who recognize that the other knows the fact but they dare not admit or discuss it openly. In their 1965 book, *Awareness of Dying,* Glaser and Strauss call this "mutual pretense awareness." It is a perfect illustration of a prominent cultural characteristic expressed in human relationships in Japan.

Building a trusting relationship between the physician and patient in Japan may very well be up to the patient. In particular, when physicians and other medical staff provide information for Japanese patients or their families, the personal relationship between the professional and patient will significantly affect the communication process. That there are many patients who want a detailed explanation of their condition from the physician but are unable to pose the kinds of questions to obtain it is clear enough. Unfortunately, without a satisfactory interpersonal relationship, constructive communication remains all too difficult.

The Family in Japan

As society ages and chronic disease morbidity rises, more and more people will have to learn to maintain a certain standard of life activities despite their existing afflictions or disabilities. Consequently, as the need for individualized care mounts, families will become more involved in playing a dominant role in healthcare. Although family members belong to a diversity of social and culture groups, only the family is concerned with the total individual and all matters related to his or her life. As Friedman (1992) points out, the family that provides for physical necessities—food, clothing, shelter, and healthcare—is the family that usually shares in the suffering and coping of the stressful health event. When a family member becomes ill, other family members give personal care, financial support, and whatever else is needed.

That universal family functions exist in healthcare is clear. That cultural differences define how families provide for healthcare is equally clear. Among Japanese, psychological support by family members plays a particularly significant role, which is explained by this peculiarity of Japanese human relationships: *the division of life into inner and outer sectors each with its own, different, standard of behavior* (Doi, 1973). Doi, a Japanese psychiatrist, states, *"since most Japanese consider it perfectly natural that a man should vary his attitude depending on whether he is dealing with his inner circle or with others, no one considers it hypocritical or contradictory that he should behave willfully within his own circle yet control himself outside it."* For most Japanese, the family remains within the most intimate circle. Besides, it takes a fairly long time before a family accepts an unrelated person or stranger. Then, as Japanese believe that we should control ourselves outside the circle—where the others are—we need to depend more upon families within our own circle for psychological matters.

Moreover, Japan has a peculiar family system in which the concept of "ie" prevails. The term "ie" also has implications beyond those to be found in the English words "household" or "family," for example (Nakane, 1984). Nakane, a Japanese anthropologist puts it this way, *"The ie is a corporate residential group and . . . comprised of household members (in most cases the family members of the household head, but others in addition to family members may be included), who thus make up the units of a distinguishable social group."* She goes on to say, *"What is important here is that the human relationships within this household group are thought of as more important than all other human relationships. Then the wife and daughter-in-law who have come from outside have incomparably greater importance than one's own sisters and daughters, who have married and gone into other households."*

In other words, if we are to understand the Japanese family system, we should understand the family unit or family structure based on a framework of residence rather than attributes of being born of the same parents. The long-term care of a bedridden elderly patient by family caregivers clearly represents characteristics of the Japanese family system.

According to the Ministry of Health and Welfare (1997), caregivers living with bedridden elderly patients (65 years or older) rose to 86.5% while 29.5% of caregivers were "spouses of the patients' children by blood" (i.e., daughters-in-law). However characteristic these findings are, as the number of nuclear families increase in Japan, the percentage of "spouses of the elderly" who take care of him or her (28.3%) will also rise.

The institution of "ie" has caused Japanese to give less weight to kinship than other societies (e.g., those in China, India, and the United States). Japanese are inclined to think of sons and daughters who have established a separate household as belonging to another family. They visit their parents less frequently than Americans do. Many Japanese also have not developed manners and customs by which siblings jointly assume responsibility in looking after their elderly parents. In the main, Japanese are ill-equiped to receive support from someone who is not included in the corporate residential group. For that reason alone, family members feel obliged to assume a good part of the responsibility, even when the health problem is far greater than he or she can manage.

Public Services for a Japanese Family

Most Japanese recognize the importance of family responsibility in long-term care. The Division of Policy Planning and Evaluation at the Ministry of Health and Welfare (1997) pooled 1995 responses to the following hypothetical question: "If an elderly member of one's household requires long-term care, how will the other members cope with it?" Subsequently, 56.5% of all respondents answered "mainly family and kinfolk attend to the elderly, perhaps aided by home welfare services" while 19.8% stated that "family and kinfolk attend to the elderly." "We rely mainly on home welfare services" or "we place the elderly in an institution" were given by 11.5% of respondents.

The results cited above offer a reflection of the Japanese mindset that prefers family members remain together at home. The results of the next survey by the Management and Coordination Agency also illustrates the same tendency. In a comparison of attitudes of the elderly (60 years or older) in various countries and their relationship with family members in 1990 (Ministry of Health and Welfare, 1996b), responses indicated that the percentage of the elderly who prefer to continue to live with their children and grandchildren was 53.6% in Japan. The figure ranked next to that from Korea, while in Western nations it was remarkably low (particularly in the United States at 3.4%). In Asian nations, it is customary for the elderly to live together with their children and grandchildren; Japan is no exception. What is uniquely Japanese, however, is the way in which Japanese accept and deal with social services provided as home care.

The 1995 data on caregivers for the bedridden elderly indicate that one-half of key caregivers were 60 years or older (Ministry of Health and Welfare, 1997). According to yet another survey conducted by the Policy Planning and Evaluation Division (Ministry of Health and Welfare, 1997) in 1995 on key and subordinate caregivers who provide long-term care at home, 38.9% of caregivers received no help from others in taking care of elderly family members, while 46.4% were assisted by subordinate caregivers, such as biological children or spouses of the children in most instances. Another outstanding finding here concerned subordinate caregivers, which included very few supporters such as neighbors or volunteers. Public service providers such as the home helper service or visiting nurse service, on the other hand, have been utilized frequently. The results suggest that while social services should be expanded, the cultural implication that overall few Japanese make use of social services is also important to consider.

Most Japanese actively seek out and consult a physician and yet are passive in receiving health and welfare services. All Japanese citizens are entitled to receive the benefits of medical insurance when the services provided fall within the prescribed medical category. On the other hand, Japanese cannot take advantage of welfare services until they request them. As Japanese are rather sensitive about behaving differently from the general public, it becomes problematic to accept public welfare service benefits.

Of course, if public services are expanded much more in the community, Japanese may then view it as more readily available. But there is yet another barrier to the availability of public services. Not all that fond of having unrelated persons or strangers, such as home helpers and visiting nurses, enter the household, Japanese tend to regard it negatively as an interference by outsiders. To the Japanese, group consciousness is commonly intense to the point where the individual's every problem must be solved within the group's framework (Nakane, 1984). Simply, most Japanese prefer to solve family members' problems such as long-term care for the elderly within their household on their own. If the home helper and the visiting nurses want to attend the family more effectively, they have to be recognized in some way as members of the household group by family members.

STRATEGIES FOR FUTURE NURSING

Although the Japanese healthcare administration system has been altered to suit national healthcare needs, the result of the alteration is more readily seen in the quality of services actually implemented. Once needs are diversified and the goal of healthcare includes not only prevention of diseases but also enjoyment of the quality of life, it is necessary to provide services in an individualized manner and at a location where recipients expect to receive them. When these goals are achieved, health providers will be engaged in actual work and provide health services. High quality nursing intervention will meet individual needs.

At medical institutions, nursing personnel have the best opportunity to interact with patients. In long-term and home-visit nursing care, they can also find larger roles in the community. In 1994 in Japan, the nurse population totaled: public health nurses (PHNs), 29,008; midwives, 23,048; registered nurses (RNs), 49,232; and assistant nurses, 369,661. Among them, 95.0% of nursing personnel were employed in hospitals or clinics, and 0.2% engaged in public healthcare as PHNs. The ratios of RNs and assistant nurses to that of PHNs per 100,000 people were 689.4 and 23.2, respectively (Ministry of Health and Welfare, 1996b). Although the number of PHNs is gradually increasing, it is not sufficient for a society where its population is aging fast.

Coping with these problems requires that a large number of highly trained nursing staff be maintained. Improvements in nursing education, which enable nurses to practice quality care, will also permit them to play a more substantial healthcare role. During the past few years, the opening of several new nursing colleges and the establishment of nursing departments in existing colleges or universities have begun to address nursing's educational needs. As of April 1994, the number of 4-year nursing colleges has reached 30, and the number of junior colleges (excluding 2-year programs) has increased to 60.

The state of affairs in healthcare has been changing in Japan. People require health services beyond the cure and prevention of disease. Nurses frequently encounter cases where they can practice care and apply their own decision-making process in patient care. Through wholesome relationships with individuals and the family, nurses should be able to provide personal care and necessary information so that the family autonomy and the patient well-being are maximized. The role of nurses is particularly important in home care in an environment where the family resides. I believe that in Japan, with the described cultural peculiarity of human relationships, it is Japanese nurses who can understand fully the needs of individuals and family, and act thereby as an important intermediary between healthcare providers and their recipients.

REFERENCES

Ashworth, P. D., Longmate, M. A., & Morrison, M. (1992). Patient participation: Its meaning and significance in the context of caring. *Journal of Advanced Nursing, 17,* 1430–1439.

Chao, Yu-Mai (1992). A unique concept of nursing care. *International Nursing Review, 39*(6), 181–184.

Doi, T. (1973). *"Amae no kozo"* The anatomy of dependence. J. Bester (Ed.), Codansha International Ltd.

Friedman, M. M. (1992). Family nursing: Theory and practice. Appleton and Lange.

Furuich, K. (Ed.). (1995). *Eisei gyousei taiyo* (16th rev. ed.). Japan Public Health Association.

Glaser, B. G., & Strauss, A. L. (1965). *Awareness of dying.* Chicago: Aldine Publishing.

Ministry of Health and Welfare of Japan (Ed.). (1996a). Annual Report on Health and Welfare 1994–1995—Medical Care—Quality, information, choice and assent. Japan International Corporation of Welfare Services.

Ministry of Health and Welfare of Japan. (Ed.). (1996b). *Annual Report on Health and Welfare 1995-1996: Family and social security—for social support to family.* Gyosei.

Nakahara, T., & Shobayashi, T. (1995). *Public health in Japan-health service systems.* Japan Public Health Association.

Nakane, C. (1984). *Japanese society.* Tokyo: Charles E. Tuttle.

Okaya, K. (1988). The study of coping style of pre-operational patients and post-operational patients. *The Japanese Journal of Nursing Research, 21*(3), 53–60.

Orimo, H. (Ed.). (1992). *Gerontology: Overview and perspectives.* Tokyo: University of Tokyo Press.

Policy Planning and Evaluation Div. at Minister's Secretariat, Ministry of Health and Welfare. (1997). Report on the General Survey of Family Function.

Population Projections for Japan by Ministry of Health and Welfare. (1992). *Population Projections for Japan; 1991-2090,* (printing).

Shibata, H. (1990). Arterioscleroses in Japanese: Epidemiological inquiry. *Gendai Iryo, 22,* 1083–1087.

Statistics and Information Department at Minister's Secretariat, Ministry of Health and Welfare. (1995a). *Patients survey.* Health and Welfare Statistics Association.

Statistics and Information Department at Minister's Secretariat, Ministry of Health and Welfare. (1995b). *Report on health service administration (Eisei Gyousei Gyomu Houkoku): 1994.* Health and Welfare Statistics Association.

Statistics and Information Department at Minister's Secretariat, Ministry of Health and Welfare. (1996a). *Vital statistics of Japan; 1994.* Health and Welfare Statistics Association.

Statistics and Information Department at Minister's Secretariat, Ministry of Health and Welfare. (1996b). *Comprehensive survey of the living conditions of people on health and welfare: 1994.* Health and Welfare Statistics Association.

Statistics and Information Department at Minister's Secretariat, Ministry of Health and Welfare. (1996c). *Survey of medical care institutions—Hospital reports: 1994.* Health and Welfare Statistics Association.

Statistics and Information Department at Minister's Secretariat, Ministry of Health and Welfare. (1996d). *National health expenditure: 1994.* Health and Welfare Statistics Association.

Statistics and Information Department at Minister's Secretariat, Ministry of Health and Welfare. (1996e). *Report on the socioeconomic survey of vital statistics—Medical treatment for the terminally ill patient: FY1994.* Health and Welfare Statistics Association.

Statistics and Information Department at Minister's Secretariat, Ministry of Health and Welfare. (1997). *Comprehensive survey of the living conditions of people on health and welfare, 1995.* Health and Welfare Statistics Association.

PART III

Education

The Use of Problem-Based Learning Tutorials with a Predominately Asian American Nursing Student Population

Dianne N. Ishida, PhD, RN

*T*he use of collaborative peer learning in educational settings as a way to assist students has been gaining momentum in the health professions. Problem-based learning (PBL), a distinctive form for collaborative peer learning, is being used in schools of medicine (Albanese & Mitchell, 1993; Berstein, Tipping, Bercovitz, & Skinner, 1995; Donner & Bickley, 1993; Vernon, 1995; Walton & Matthews, 1989; Woodward & Ferrier, 1983) and, more recently, in schools of nursing (Andrews & Jones, 1996; Cerny, Amundson, Mueller, & Waldron, 1996; Creedy & Hand, 1994; Creedy, Horsfall, & Hand, 1992; Ishida, 1995; Little & Ryan, 1988). Although PBL literature focuses on effective methods and tutoring (faculty) receptiveness and training (Berstein et al., 1995; Davis, Nairn, Paine, Anderson, & Oh, 1992; Des Marchais, Bureau, Dumais, & Pigeon, 1992; Dolmans, Gijselaers, Schmidt, & Van Der Meer, 1993; Kaufman & Mann, 1996; Mayo, Donnelly, & Schwartz, 1995; Vasconez, Donnelly, Mayo, & Schwartz, 1993; Vernon, 1995; Vernon & Blake, 1993), it has failed to address multiethnic student population contexts, particularly with those ethnic groups (e.g., Asian Americans) that tend to be culturally less verbal. As our nation and our universities become more multiethnic, however, educators need to consider how teaching approaches affect the learning of all cultural groups.

PROBLEM-BASED LEARNING LITERATURE

Although problem-based learning appeared initially in the Socratic dia-
logues and remained a part of medical education in the form of bedside
clinical teaching, its most current form—PBL—originated at McMaster
University School of Medicine in Ontario in the late 1960s. Since then, it
has spread throughout North America, and is practiced in such institutions as Michigan State University, the University of New Mexico, Harvard, the University of Sherbrooke in Quebec, the University of Hawaii
(Albanese & Mitchell, 1993), the University of Kentucky (Vasconez et al.,
1993), and Mercer University (Donner & Bickley, 1993). PBL also has
spread around the world, to the University of Limburg in The Netherlands
(Dolmans et al., 1993) and the Clinical School in Wellington, New
Zealand (Lewis, Buckley, Kong, & Mellsop, 1992).

In an era of rapid information growth, technological advances, and
attention to individuality, the traditional medical education (2 years of
discipline-based basic science lectures followed by 2 years of clinical
clerkships) is perceived as dehumanizing, demotivating, inefficient, and
even ineffective. Recognizing these deficiencies, the founding fathers of
McMaster University School of Medicine responded in kind. Medical education, or so they felt, should be fun—students learn best when actively
involved; basic science concepts are understood and remembered when
presented in a clinically relevant format (Neufeld & Barrows, 1974).

The theoretical underpinnings of PBL include using prior knowledge to
understand and structure new information, encoding specificity (context)
to make the transfer of learning more likely as it reflects real-life situations
encountered in practice, and the elaborating on knowledge through discussing, answering questions, peer teaching, and critiquing (Schmidt,
1983). Peers serve as more knowledgeable individuals after completing
their research on specific group-selected learning issues. Faculty serve as
tutors who facilitate the process, assisting students to problem solve, explore all relevant issues sufficiently, and critique the information presented
(Barrows, 1988).

At its fundamental level, PBL is an instructional approach characterized by the use of patient problems as a context for developing students'
problem-solving skills and acquiring basic and clinical science knowledge
(Albanese & Mitchell, 1993). The PBL process involves students meeting
in small groups (generally 5–6 in number) with an assigned tutor for the
full semester. Students are presented with a real-life problem, situation,
or simulation that is ill-structured in the same way actual problems present themselves to health professionals, that is, without all the needed information for proper evaluation.

In order to manage the problem effectively, students use a hypothetico-deductive process to determine the information needed to understand the nature of the problem and its possible causes (Barrows, 1988). A number of hypotheses are generated to guide the inquiry, to guide the type and sequence of inquiries that need to be made (i.e., questions, probes, observations, examinations). Once the group has generated a list of learning issues (what the group needs to know) to manage the problem, the members divide the work for individual research. Students may be provided with lists of resources such as agencies, faculty, textbooks, and videotapes. At the group's next meeting, students report, as more knowledgeable peers, their research. They discuss their findings and develop a shared understanding of the client's situation; this then allows them to determine a plan of care to manage the patient effectively.

The PBL process ideally includes evaluating the information resources utilized, analyzing how students could have better managed the patient's problem, and critiquing one's own and the group's performance. This important aspect may be overlooked as students become more involved in the technical or pathophysiological processes of the patient's condition. Part of the tutor's responsibility is allotting time for evaluation of the tutorial sessions.

Though the criteria to judge the outcomes of PBL have not been universally agreed upon, the strengths and weaknesses of PBL have been noted in the literature. Experimental design weaknesses have been recognized in the studying of curricular innovations (Albanese & Mitchell, 1993). Yet the cited strengths of PBL are many. Questionnaires sent to PBL tutors at 22 U.S. and Canadian medical schools revealed that respondents evaluated PBL more positively than traditional methods. This was particularly evident in student interest and enthusiasm, faculty interest and enthusiasm, tutor satisfaction, and student reasoning and preparation for clinical rotations (Vernon, 1995). PBL and the traditional methods, however, were judged equally efficient for learning.

THE EFFECTIVENESS OF PROBLEM-BASED LEARNING

A study at the University of Toronto Faculty of Medicine similarly noted that direct experience with PBL led to more favorable attitudes among students and faculty (Berstein et al., 1995). Students said PBL improved teamwork and doctor-patient relationships. They found PBL stimulating and enjoyable and believed it taught them how to learn rather than to memorize These sentiments were reinforced at Georgia's Mercer University School of

Medicine, where most faculty favored the PBL curriculum over conventional curricula because it seems a "more natural format for learning" and contains built-in motivational features (Donner & Bickley, 1993). Unless a student carefully prepared for tutorials, other group members complained loudly. In contrast to a lecture-based program, where students study after class, PBL students routinely spent 5 to 8 hours preparing for each tutorial. Students learned to utilize a wide variety of resources and then reconcile in their group discussions conflicting information from different resources. This promoted the development of critical thinking skills. Also, since it promoted better student-faculty relationships, students perceived the PBL curriculum as more egalitarian than conventional curricula.

PBL students demonstrated significantly deeper learning and less surface learning than traditional medical school students (Newble & Clark, 1986). They showed greater conceptualization and less memorization, and they judged new information more critically (Moore, Block, & Mitchell, 1990). The PBL learning environment encouraged an inquisitive style of learning rather than rote learning (Schmidt, Dauphinee, & Patel, 1987), creating a usable body of knowledge in the students' minds. The physician skills important for patients are problem solving skills, not memory skills (Barrows & Tamblyn, 1980). An equally important strength of PBL was the development of skills and motivation required for continued self-directed learning and self-assessment skills in the practice context (Walton & Matthews, 1989).

The weaknesses of PBL have primarily focused on national examination results and gaps in knowledge. Medical students in some instances scored lower on basic science examinations and viewed themselves as less capable in the basic sciences (National Board of Medical Examiners–Part I) than the traditionally prepared students (Albanese & Mitchell, 1993). This was reinforced by Vernon's (1995) data in which traditional methods were judged to be superior for teaching factual knowledge of basic sciences. However, PBL students were perceived to have performed better on clinical examinations (National Board of Medical Examiners–Parts II and III) (Albanese & Mitchell, 1993). An expressed concern was the appropriateness of the traditional paper-and-pencil measurement, like the examinations of the National Board of Medical Examiners, a tool for evaluating PBL program outcomes, which are more process oriented.

A perceived student concern is that PBL may result in knowledge gaps or reinforcement of incorrect information (Berstein et al., 1995). Structuring the range of context available into a set number of PBL cases may achieve more depth and knowledge in some areas at the cost of less or minimal knowledge in other areas. Various schools and faculty have handled these concerns in a variety of ways: adding selected resources or lectures, reconfiguring cases to cover gaps, and reemphasizing student critiquing of presented information to correct inaccuracies.

A related concern is the variability to tutor quality (Donner & Bickley, 1993). Discussion and research has centered around whether the tutor is a content expert or not. Ideally, the tutor is both an expert tutor and expert in the discipline under study (Barrows, 1988), but this combination has not been feasible in schools of medicine. Tutors who have good facilitator skills can assist the group to work through its case problems. However, students generally perceive higher tutor effectiveness if the tutor has thorough, up-to-date knowledge of the problem under study or if the tutor is seen as a clinical expert (Feletti, Dole, Petrovic, & Sanson-Fisher, 1982). Expert content tutors tend to be more directive and less facilitative than noncontent experts, a situation which could inhibit students from introducing their own ideas (Davis et al., 1992). This, however, is not supported by a study by Eagle, Harasym, and Mandin (1992). Students with clinically expert tutors identified twice as many learning issues (areas to explore) and spent almost twice as much time studying for the case, than did students with nonexpert content tutors. Also, the learning issues identified by the expert tutor groups were almost three times as likely to be congruent with case objectives than their nonexpert counterparts. Patel, Groen, and Norman (1991) suggested that the higher error rate on clinical care problems of PBL students compared to conventional students may occur because nonexpert tutors perpetuate misconceptions by leaving errors uncorrected.

High resource utilization (i.e., faculty time, library, and other resources) is another concern of PBL curriculum (Albanese & Mitchell, 1993; Donner & Bickley, 1993). Much faculty time is required for curriculum development, especially to assure that essential content areas are covered by the selected cases. Decisions were needed on the breadth and depth of content and the degree of complexity appropriate for each case. Interdisciplinary input needs to be coordinated with faculty from the basic natural and social sciences, as well as the clinical specialities. Library and other resources need to be in place. Faculty commitment is needed to implement the change in pedagogy, requiring faculty to acquire tutorials skills essential to the process (Creedy, Horsfall, & Hand, 1992). Curriculum implementation also entails heavy faculty utilization, since faculty to student-tutorial ratios are generally much smaller than those of large lecture classes.

Revising a complete curriculum is a time-consuming process and sometimes costly, but at Sherbrooke School of Medicine in Quebec, the shift from a traditional to a PBL curriculum was made without additional financial resources. It, however, severely taxed the teachers' available resources (Des Marchais et al., 1992). Comparing costs of maintaining PBL and conventional curricula depends on many factors: faculty and student time commitments, personnel-support requirements, instruction materials, necessary physical support (e.g., small rooms), and so forth. Once implemented, faculty effort in the two curricula (PBL and conventional) may not differ much in terms of time per week, but may differ in how the time is spent. Conventional track teachers spend more time preparing and less time teaching compared to PBL faculty, who spend more time in direct teaching (Albanese & Mitchell, 1993). Lewis and Tamblyn (1987) also noted that cost and preparation time on the part of instructors is "not a significant issue" when comparing an experimental PBL group to a conventional control group within a senior baccalaureate nursing class.

In two summary articles (Berkson, 1993; Norman & Schmidt, 1992), there were small or little differences between the overall knowledge or competence of medical students trained by PBL and those from conventional curricula. It was difficult to distinguish one set of graduates from the other. Most students were flexible in their choice of learning strategy and were capable in utilizing comprehensive-directed approaches, as well as strategic rote-learning behavior. What was important was the feedback mechanism that is generally a part of the PBL approach.

A similar result was found with nursing students. In a study of the PBL in a baccalaureate nursing program, Lewis and Tamblyn (1987) found no significant difference in measurable theoretical or problem solving outcomes between the PBL senior nursing group and its traditional lecture counterpart. However, the PBL group reported more willingness to learn and with greater depth than they previously did with a lecture format.

Overall, the strengths in a PBL curriculum include motivational factors for student and faculty, utilization of self-directed learning strategies important for life-long learning, a focus on real-life situations encountered in the profession, a greater depth and retention of information, and the facilitation of cognitive processes that support clinical reasoning and thinking.

STUDY SETTING AND SAMPLE

Much of the material discussed in this chapter was gleaned from a department of nursing study that included ethnically diverse students and faculty. The undergraduate baccalaureate class that was studied reflected this diversity. In the class of 34, there were 7 of mixed ethnicity, 7 Caucasians, and 20 Asian Americans. The Asian Americans included, in descending order, 13 Filipinos, 4 Japanese, and 1 Chinese, 1 Korean, and 1 Vietnamese student. When asked with what cultural groups they identified, most students selected their own ethnic group, using terms as "Filipino American" or "Japanese American." A few used terms such as "local" or "Midwesterner." As a result, the students citing ethnicity were used for the study. All students were female and had a median age of 23.2 years. They ranged from first generation (foreign born) to fourth generation and beyond. The bulk of the students were either second or third generation. Half of the class participated in a questionnaire at the end of the second semester. The questionnaire included information on the subject's sociocultural context for learning and how he or she processed new information. Asian participants consisted of approximately half the primary ethnic groups in the nursing class. The total number of Asian students comprised 59% of this sample. Additionally, there were 3 Caucasian students and 4 students of part-Asian ethnicity who were placed in a mixed ethnic category. The nursing class was tracked through graduation. A follow-up interview was conducted at the end of the final semester with 12 students, half of whom were of Asian ethnicity. The interview focused on what teaching modalities in the program helped the student learn and what could be improved upon. The data discussed was derived primarily from the questionnaire and interview.

The department of nursing in this study adopted a broadly defined inquiry-based learning (IBL) philosophy that considered students and faculty as co-learners with student-driven learning experiences to achieve the goals of nursing practice. Students were actively involved and assumed responsibility for their learning while faculty guided and facilitated the learning process. Various teaching modalities have been incorporated into this IBL philosophy, such as PBL tutorials, lectures, discussions, laboratories, and group work.

PBL Tutorials

At the time of the study, the PBL tutorials were pervasive in the nursing curriculum, being utilized in most of the clinical courses after the first semester. These tutorials were patterned after the PBL tutorials of Barrows (1988). Each tutorial group consisted of a clinical group (8–10 students)

with a clinical faculty member serving as the tutor with content expertise. Interaction was enhanced by sitting around a table in a room with a
blackboard or large writing tablets. The cases discussed in the tutorials
generally were predesigned by the faculty teaching the course to ensure
adequate coverage of relevant concepts. In the final semester, the clinical
courses utilized the students' real clients as cases in the tutorials. The
case was revealed to the students in a sequential manner during the first
tutorial session, simulating what would occur in a real clinical situation.
Students discussed what was known about the situation and generated
hypotheses, which are then written on the board. The tutor's role at this
stage was to keep students on track and to encourage them to explore all
relevant issues and questions and think critically about the cases under
discussion. If an important issue was not addressed, the tutor would ask
students if there were other areas to explore. Once students determined
what they needed to know about the case (learning issues), they divided
areas of research among themselves.

At the next session, students shared and discussed their research findings. Questions about each other's data and sources of information were
encouraged to prevent misinterpretations or errors and facilitate understanding. When necessary, the tutor questioned students to promote thinking and problem solving. To facilitate the presentations, students generally
wrote their findings for the group members. After sharing their research,
students discussed and identified client needs and approaches to meet
those needs, which were then written on the board.

Within the tutorials, some tutors were more active than others; ideally
they did not lecture or dominate the discussions, but remained in the
background and facilitated the process. The tutors monitored the sessions
to see that all relevant learning issues were discussed sufficiently. Each
session included time allotted to process how the group evaluated its past
performance and how the sessions could be improved; any interpersonal
conflicts were resolved at this time. The tutor helped the group set
ground rules for the tutorials and determine individual tasks for members
(e.g., recorder, case facilitator, timekeeper, etc.).

Information Processing

Students were asked to describe how they processed new information. This
was done narratively by students without cues from the researcher. Students indicated multiple ways of processing new information. However,

interacting with others was the response most frequently mentioned by the 17 students who completed the questionnaire. Eighty-eight percent (15 of the 17 students) indicated that they process new information by interacting with others. Students noted they found it helpful to discuss and exchange ideas with others.

Seventy-six percent (13 students) selected visualization and application as popular methods used to process new information. Student responses coded as visualization consisted of highlighting important information, outlining, diagraming, using flowcharts, seeing, and writing. Responses such as "hands on" were coded as application. Seventy percent of the Asian students interviewed mentioned visualization and 60% mentioned application, while 75% of the Caucasian students mentioned visualization and all mentioned application as ways to process new information. All the part-Asian mixed ethnic students selected both visualization and application.

Interestingly, these top three methods students said they used to process new information are all part of the PBL process.

Teaching Modalities—What Aided Learning

Within the nursing school, students were exposed to various teaching modalities including lectures, seminars, PBL tutorials, group projects and presentations, and other group work. The PBL tutorials were pervasive in at least one clinical course per semester in three of the four semesters in the undergraduate program.

With few exceptions, most students had occasional group experience prior to nursing school, but these were mostly in extracurricular activities such as sports, clubs, and school committees. The predominant experience in the classroom was the traditional teacher-driven didactic lecture approach. For most students, the nursing school's PBL tutorial was a new experience.

When students were asked what helped them to learn, they consistently referred to the PBL tutorials and clinical. This was consistent with two of the ways students stated they processed new information—interaction and application. Students from various ethnic groups remarked that they liked working with the "real cases," an assignment implemented in the last semester of clinical tutorials. As an Asian student shared, "Working with real case [I] had to go back to implement . . . [I] worked harder . . . looking for resources had meaning. . . . [I] could evaluate the care."

Students overwhelmingly indicated that the PBL tutorials as a teaching approach helped them to learn. With one exception, the few students who did not like the PBL tutorials at the end of the second semester of the program revised their opinion by the program's end. The comment from two Asian students in this group was that PBL was a new experience for them, unlike the more familiar lectures.

Nursing students of all ethnic groups seem to find PBL facilitated their learning. The following were comments elicited from the interviews at the end of the program. Students remarked on the importance of being actively engaged in the learning process—deciding their own learning issues, researching them, and discussing them with peers. A part-Asian/Hawaiian/Caucasian student noted how peers were "sparking off" each other to come up with "more good ideas." One Asian student said she tried to have study or peer discussions outside of class, too; she felt PBL was a "model for practice—consultation." A part-Asian student noted, "You have all these people to consult, your peers." Another part-Asian student stated, "Peers could relate it [to you] in a way you could understand." She and other students liked suggesting learning issues on "what we think is important." An Asian student remarked that she retained information better through PBL because "you are actively learning it yourself" and "you have to understand to present it [to your peers]." She noted further that "it's natural now, if you don't know, you seek the information out."

Another aspect of PBL tutorials is that they help build relationships among students and between student and faculty. This seemed particularly important to the Asian students. One Asian student in particular remarked that PBL was a positive school experience:

> Not because it is a good way to learn (although it is) because of the way it fosters group relationship; never have I worked so cooperatively with a group. I feel they can relate to everything I have been thinking and feeling while in nursing school. Together we have learned so much in such a little time and have become good friends through the experience.

The PBL tutorial created a small group atmosphere in which quieter, culturally hesitant students like the Asian American students felt comfortable to participate. A few students noted that they felt comfortable to speak up and that tutorials could even motivate the quieter ones to speak. As the students began to know one another better, they generally began to work together as a group, developing trust and becoming more cohesive. It became easier for even the quiet ones to take initiative and participate. The sharing of individual research findings provided one clear avenue for participation in the tutorials. An Asian student of Filipino ancestry noted that the quiet students would talk if asked directly, "What do you think?" This is supported by Chattergy and Ongteco (1991) who noted that Filipino students preferred to be called on or "nominated" by the teacher rather than to volunteer a response. The "rightness" or "wrongness" of the response was, thus, placed on the teacher (not the student), lessening the embarrassment of the student for a wrong answer. When active participation was expected, Filipino students preferred smaller classes in which one-to-one interactions and more personal relationships with instructors were possible (Castillo & Minamishin, 1991). A Filipino student noted that the "relationship with the instructor really makes a difference—if the relationship is good, I tend to do better." The tutorial format provided the setting and atmosphere for relationships to form.

Student recommendations for the PBL tutorials were elicited. Most centered on defining role expectations of faculty and student in the tutorials. The initial orientation of students (and faculty) to PBL was crucial. This led faculty to the development of mock cases for demonstration and two videotapes to demonstrate the features of the tutorials and the roles of tutor and student (Chase & Flannelly, 1993; Flannelly & Chase, 1993). Faculty in each class should review role expectations at the beginning of each course and periodically as needed. In the initial PBL courses or sessions, faculty may need to be more directive and role model the behaviors expected until students become accustomed to the tutorials. Faculty should clarify to what extent they plan to participate in the tutorials. Students from all cultural groups said they needed feedback to ensure they were on track in the tutorials. Most students wanted tutor intervention if there was misinformation, if key issues were being overlooked or incompletely covered, and if there were problems within the group. The regular evaluation of the tutorial session was crucial in resolving group member problems. As one Asian student noted, "You don't want to hurt their feelings . . . [so] make generalized statements not to pin point out the person." This student would make general statements rather than confront a peer during the group processing of the sessions. Asian Americans generally prefer to maintain group harmony and avoid conflict (Chang, 1981, 1995; Ishida & Inouye, 1995; Vance, 1995). The Asian students tended to value and work to maintain group harmony and relationships with peers.

The depth and breadth of individual student research and time constraints were other key concerns. Some students were overwhelmed with the amount of information they could uncover on their learning issue, while others just searched their textbooks. Faculty and students have handled these issues in various ways, and they should be discussed as a group. Faculty may specify a number of outside sources or research articles for each report or may provide a resource list from which students are expected to search or assign grades to research presentations. Limiting presentations to a set time with written handouts and references was one way this dilemma was handled. A Caucasian student noted that PBL saved her time since she had to research only one issue rather than all of them. As students became comfortable with PBL, they created ground rules for their tutorials. For instance, if a student report had insufficient depth or coverage, he or she was asked for a written follow-up within a specified time period. Students' roles thus emerged in some tutorials—case facilitator, recorder, and timekeeper.

A few Asian students suggested having occasional lectures accompany the tutorials. While expressing how much she liked to do research for tutorials, a Filipino student said lectures were "helpful to cover a lot when teachers emphasize what is important in an area, what problems could occur, and what to watch out for." Another Filipino student expressed a similar concern about not covering the breadth of material needed since "[we] can't cover much material with cases." Most students, however, preferred not returning to lecture-only classes again. Various courses have since added a mixture of resources including lectures with the tutorials to fill in the gaps not covered by the cases.

Other recommendations could be gleaned from the one Caucasian student who consistently did not like PBL. She felt that different instructors expected different things and some provided more guidance. She noted that different things (discussions) occurred in different groups. She felt she could not rely on her peers to present "thorough information." The student felt some students used only the textbook since some courses only tested from the textbook. Also, she felt her questions were not answered. The clarification of tutor role and the extent of participation by the tutor could help remedy the situation. Each faculty tutor is an individual and, thus, may vary somewhat on how he or she handles the tutorials. Initially, tutor workshops were made available for faculty; *The Tutorial Process* by Barrows (1988) was the primary text for these workshops. Faculty may need to continue discussions among themselves on the tutor role. Paying attention to assure all learning issues and questions are handled is also important.

Limitations of the Study

The small sample and varying number of each ethnic grouping was a limitation. The Filipinos were the largest Asian group and, thus, had more discernible patterns. While all the students who completed the questionnaire and graduated with the class were interviewed, only two students did not wish to be interviewed. The remaining three students had decelerated in the program and did not graduate with their class. Another limitation was that students did not always provide complete data, and some questions were altogether not addressed.

IMPLICATIONS FOR EDUCATION

The study clearly supports collaborative learning approaches, such as PBL, to facilitate the learning of nursing students of various cultural groups, particularly those from Asian backgrounds. Early cultivation of relationships and clarification of roles is crucial. Introductory exercises that serve as ice breakers and provide valuable understanding of students' backgrounds, prior experiences, and areas of expertise help to establish groundwork for future linkages between tutorial group members.

The ability of the tutor to facilitate the groups, knowing when to let them work independently and when to intervene, cannot be overemphasized. The role of the tutor is a paradigm shift from the traditional faculty role. No longer the main source of wisdom and knowledge, the tutor must encourage students to explore various resources and critically review them. As students learn to find answers they need for future practice, they feel more confident in themselves as practitioners. They have taken ownership of their learning, and it is hoped they will become life-long learners.

Within the tutorial groups students learn how to work together as a team and are exposed to various group conflicts and problems. These elements—teamwork and problem solving skills—are valued within the nursing profession.

In summary, the PBL tutorials assist Asian students, as well as Caucasian students, in their learning. It provides a conducive atmosphere in which peer and faculty relationships can be fostered; students can take responsibility and ownership of their learning; teamwork skills can be sharpened; and a greater depth and retention of usable knowledge can be gained. As the literature indicates, PBL is not a quick cure but involves extensive planning, an educational paradigm shift, and collaborative effort among faculty. Student feedback must continually be evaluated to assure student learning is facilitated.

REFERENCES

Albanese, M. A., & Mitchell, S. (1993). Problem-based learning: A review of literature on its outcomes and implementation issues. *Academic Medicine, 68*(1), 52–81.

Andrews, M., & Jones, P. R. (1996). Problem-based learning in an undergraduate nursing programme: A case study. *Journal of Advanced Nursing, 23*, 357–365.

Barrows, H. S. (1988). *The tutorial process.* Springfield: Southern Illinois University School of Medicine.

Berkson, L. (1993). Problem-based learning: Have the expectations been met? *Academic Medicine, 68*(10), S79–S88.

Berstein, P., Tipping, J., Bercovitz, K., & Skinner, H. A. (1995). Shifting students and faculty to a PBL curriculum: Attitudes changed and lessons learned. *Academic Medicine, 70*(3), 245–247.

Castillo, C. A., & Minamishin, S. B. (1991). Filipino recruitment and retention at the University of Hawai'i at Manoa, Honolulu. *Social Process in Hawaii, 33*, 130–141.

Cerny, J. E., Amundson, M. J., Mueller, C. W., & Waldron, J. A. (1996). Inquiry based learning, nursing student attitudes and the HIV patient. *Journal of Nursing Education, 35*(5), 219–222.

Chang, B. (1981). Asian-American patient care. In G. Henderson & M. Primeaux (Eds.), *Transcultural health care* (pp. 255–278). Menlo Park, CA: Addison-Wesley.

Chang, K. (1995). Chinese Americans. In J. N. Giger & R. E. Davidhizar (Eds.), *Transcultural nursing: Assessment and intervention* (2nd ed., pp. 395–414). St. Louis, MO: Mosby.

Chase, L., & Flannelly, L. (1993). *Strategies of small group tutorials: Roles and responsibilities of students and tutor* [Videotape]. Honolulu: University of Hawaii at Manoa.

Chattergy, V., & Ongteco, B. C. (1991). Education needs of Filipino migrant students. *Social Process in Hawaii, 33*, 142–152.

Creedy, D., & Hand, B. (1994). The implementation of problem-based learning: changing pedagogy in nurse education. *Journal of Advanced Nursing, 20*, 696–702.

Creedy, D., Horsfall, J., & Hand, B. (1992). Problem based learning in nursing education: An Australian view. *Journal of Advanced Nursing, 17*, 727–733.

Davis, W. K., Nairn, R., Paine, M. E., Anderson, R. M., & Oh, M. S. (1992). Effects of expert and non-expert facilitators on the small-group process and on student performance. *Academic Medicine, 67*, 470–474.

Des Marchais, J. E., Bureau, M. A., Dumais, B., & Pigeon, G. (1992). From traditional to problem-based learning: A case report of complete curriculum reform. *Medical Education, 16,* 190–199.

Dolmans, D. H., Gijselaers, W. H., Schmidt, H. G., & Van Der Meer, S. B. (1993).
Problem effectiveness in a course using problem-based learning. *Academic
Medicine, 68*(3), 207–213.

Donner, R. S., & Bickley, H. (1993). Problem-based learning in American medical
education: An overview. *Bulletin of the Medical Library Association, 81*(3),
294–298.

Eagle, C. J., Harasym, P. H., & Mandin, H. (1992). Effects of tutors with case expertise on problem-based learning issues. *Academic Medicine, 67,* 465–469.

Feletti, G. I., Doyle, E., Petrovic, A., & Sanson-Fisher, R. (1982). Medical students'
evaluation of tutors in a group-learning curriculum. *Medical Education, 16,*
319–325.

Flannelly, L., & Chase, L. (1993). *Strategies of small group tutorials: Introduction to basic features of small group tutorials* [Videotape]. Honolulu: University of Hawaii at Manoa.

Ishida, D., & Inouye, J. (1995). Japanese Americans. In J. N. Giger & R. E. Davidhizar (Eds.), *Transcultural nursing: Assessment and intervention* (2nd ed.,
pp. 317–345). St. Louis, MO: Mosby.

Ishida, D. N. (1995). Learning preferences among ethnically diverse nursing
students exposed to a variety of collaborative learning approaches including problem-based learning (Doctoral Dissertation, University of Hawaii at
Manoa). *UMI's Dissertation Abstracts, 2767.*

Kaufman, D. M., & Mann, K. V. (1996). Comparing students' attitudes in problem-
based and conventional curricula. *Academic Medicine, 71*(10), 1096–1099.

Lewis, K. E., & Tamblyn, R. M. (1987). The problem-based learning approach in
baccalaureate nursing education: How effective is it? *Nursing Papers/Per-
spectives in Nursing, 19*(2), 17–26.

Lewis, M. E., Buckley, A., Kong, M., & Mellsop, G. W. (1992). The role of evaluation in the development of a problem-based learning programme within a
traditional school of medicine. *Annual Community-Oriented Education, 5,*
223–234.

Little, P., & Ryan, G. (1988). Educational change through problem-based learning. *The Australian Journal of Advanced Nursing, 5*(4), 31–35.

Mayo, W. P., Donnelly, M. B., & Schwartz, R. W. (1995). Characteristics of the
ideal problem-based learning tutor in clinical medicine. *Evaluation and the
Health Professions, 18*(2), 124–136.

Moore, G. T., Block, S., & Mitchell, R. (1990). *A random controlled trial evaluating the impact of the new pathway curriculum at Harvard Medical
School.* Final Report to the Fund for the Improvement of Post-Secondary Education, Harvard University, Boston.

Neufeld, V. R., & Barrows, H. S. (1974). The "McMaster Philosophy": An approach to medical education. *Journal of Medical Education, 49,* 1040–1050.

Newble, D. I., & Clarke, R. M. (1986). The approach to learning of students in a traditional and an innovative problem-based medical school. *Medical Education, 20,* 267–273.

Norman, G. R., & Schmidt, G. G. (1992). The psychological basis of problem-based learning: A review of the evidence. *Academic Medicine, 76*(9), 557–565.

Patel, V. L., Groen, G. J., & Norman, G. R. (1991). Effects of conventional and problem-based medical curricula on problem solving. *Academic Medicine, 66*(7), 380–389.

Schmidt, H. G. (1983). Problem-based learning: Rationale and description. *Medical Education, 17,* 11–16.

Schmidt, H. G., Dauphinee, W. D., & Patel, V. L. (1987). Comparing the effects of problem-based learning and conventional curricula in an international sample. *Journal of Medical Education, 62*(4), 305–315.

Vance, A. R. (1995). Filipino Americans. In J. N. Giger & R. E. Davidhizar (Eds.), *Transcultural nursing: Assessment and intervention* (2nd ed., pp. 417–438). St. Louis, MO: Mosby.

Vasconez, H. C., Donnelly, M. B., Mayo, P., & Schwartz, R. W. (1993). Student perceptions of the effectiveness of a problem-based surgery curriculum. *Academic Medicine, 68*(10), S28–S30.

Vernon, D. T. (1995). Attitudes and opinions of faculty tutors about problem-based learning. *Academic Medicine, 70*(3), 216–223.

Vernon, D. T., & Blake, R. L. (1993). Does problem-based learning work? A meta-analysis of evaluative research. *Academic Medicine, 68,* 550–563.

Walton, H. J., & Matthews, M. B. (1989). Essentials of problem-based learning. *Medical Education, 23,* 542–558.

Woodward, C. A., & Ferrier, B. M. (1983). The content of the medical curriculum at McMaster University: Graduate's evaluation of their preparation for post-graduate training. *Medical Education, 17,* 54–60.

CHAPTER TWELVE

Taiwanese Nursing

Yi Chun Lo, MA, RN

*T*aiwan actually derives from two words in Chinese, *Tai* and *wan*, meaning "terraced bay." An island located east of China's south-central coast, Taiwan also is known as Republic of China (R.O.C.) or Formosa. The name *Formosa* was coined by the Dutch hundreds of years ago and means "beautiful island." Taiwan is the size of Massachusetts, Rhode Island, and Connecticut combined, and is surrounded by 15 to 20 smaller islands considered geographically linked to it. Taiwan has rainfall year round, providing the island with a source for hydroelectric power and nourishment for agriculture. Summer is hot, humid, and long, lasting from April to October. The average temperature on the island is 70° (Copper, 1996; Jeng, 1980).

THE PEOPLE

In 1995, the population numbered 21,244,000, making Taiwan one of the most densely populated places on the globe. The island's population was only 5.8 million before people fleeing from mainland China arrived after World War II in 1949. Subsequently, a high birth rate during the next 15 years caused the population to swell to over 10 million people. In order to handle the aging population (male life expectancy is 72 years; for females, 77.4), the government introduced slogans, such as: "Two is just right, one is not too few" to encourage married couples to reduce the number of childbirths in their family. Whether a result of the government program, by 1982 the birth rate had dropped to 2.34 from 4.66 per 1,000 persons in 1952 (Copper, 1996).

Taiwan includes four major ethnic groups: Aborigines, considered to be of Indonesian or Malayan origin; two groups of Taiwanese Chinese, early Chinese migrants from Fukien and Canton almost one thousand years ago, and more than 1.5 million mainlander Chinese who arrived in Taiwan from China in 1949. Each group has its own dialect. Adding to the language diversity were the Japanese who occupied Taiwan for 50 years until the end of World War II and forced many people to speak Japanese.

To facilitate communication and also decrease conflict among the different groups, the Taiwanese government encourages people to speak the same language. Mandarin has been the official language since 1949 (Copper, 1996; Jeng, 1980).

CULTURE AND EDUCATION

Culturally, the influence of China predominates, yet colonial rule by Japan and missionary activities from the West also play significant roles in Taiwanese socialization. Because the government supports Taiwanese culture, subsequently supporting Taiwanese education, education has become the country's foundation. Translating the Chinese word for education, *chiao-yu,* provides a clear picture of the importance of education in modern Taiwan: *Chiao* means "to guide, counsel, incite, teach" (Liang, 1981, p. 228). *Yu* means "to give birth; to nourish, nurse, to help grow" (Liang, 1981, p. 421).

In examining Taiwanese education, it is important to consider the influence of Confucius. As Smith (1991, p. 7) described it, "It was Confucius' view that moral behavior was governed by relations and respect . . . The basis of Confucius' educational view was that education knows no class distinction and does not therefore discriminate." At that time the first competitive examination system was established to end the nepotistic selection of China's leaders. This made it possible for civil servants to take on the responsibilities of directing the nation's institutions. This governmental competitive examination was adopted by the Taiwanese education system; moreover, the degree of government involvement increased (Harrell, Stevan, & Huang, 1994; Smith, 1991). Centralization characterizes the administrative structure of the ROC; its highest and central governing educational body is the Ministry of Education.

Taiwan's current school system was influenced by the United States. Six years of elementary education are followed by three years of junior high school, then three years of high school, and four years of a university education. Currently, education is compulsory from elementary through junior high; by the year 2000, compulsory education will include high school. Why did the government implement, in 1968, nine years of free education? Because the government discovered economic growth had placed the country in a strong financial position.

Those students who wish to go to colleges and universities in Taiwan's higher education system must take the national Joint College Entrance Examination (JCEE) given each summer. A similar examination is given to ninth-grade students who wish to be admitted to an academic high school or vocational school. All of these examinations are given by the Ministry of Education. Only those students with the highest scores on the respective examinations are given first choice of school and a field of study. Others are relegated to their second choices. This process continues until all places are filled for the forthcoming school year (Hsiung, 1981).

Beyond the nine years of free education, there are two major types of high schools: vocational and academic. Higher education in Taiwan comprises junior, professional junior, and four-year degree granting colleges and universities. Among junior colleges, there are five-year, two-year, and three-year schools. And among these schools, the senior vocational schools and five-year junior colleges admit students as early as age 15.

NURSING

Education

During the nineteenth century, many missionaries came to China to build churches, schools, and hospitals. But it was Mckechnie from the United States, who in 1884 introduced the Nightingale Model to nursing schools in China. These schools aimed to train hospital nurses and instruct them in the training of others. In 1909, the Nurses' Association of China (NAC) was established. Science and the art of nursing was propelled forward when the NAC was responsible for the accreditation of hospital nursing schools and licensure, which was later taken over by the Ministry of Education in 1937. The president of NAC, Mei-Yu Chou, transferred the association to Taiwan in 1949; in 1961, and during the year's annual NAC meeting, the members passed a resolution to rename the organization the Nurses' Association of the Republic of China (NAROC). It was at that moment when significant reforms in nursing education were initiated (Chu, 1988).

In 1954, Taiwan Nursing Junior College was established in Taipei, Taiwan, and it provided a registered nurse (RN) program, and was the first nursing program to admit high school graduates. In 1956, the first baccalaureate nursing program was established at National Taiwan University. Five-year junior colleges were established in many cities during 1963, and in 1979, the first master's program for nursing was established at the National Defense Medical College. This program's major goal was to produce nursing educators and administrators. Likewise, in 1984 National Taiwan University established its own master's program to focus on nursing research. In 1990, evening classes were developed for junior colleges and baccalaureate programs to allow nurses to receive higher degrees while still working during the day. In 1994, in order to improve the role and function of nurses in the healthcare system, Open University developed a distance learning program and awarded graduates with BSN degrees. By 1996, Taiwan had 17 vocational schools, 10 junior colleges, 11 baccalaureate programs, 7 master programs, and 1 doctoral program in nursing (Shen, 1995).

Until 1985, the majority of nurses graduated from senior vocational schools, entering the workforce to practice healthcare at the young ages of 18 and 19. This caused a major impact in the nursing professional structure. According to 1992 data from the Department of Health, the nurse turnover rate was between 15% and 40%, the major reason being a lack of organizational commitment, which included the following factors: family, shift schedule (especially the night shift), and lack of opportunities for advancement. The average salary for an RN with 5 to 9 years experience was between NT$35,000 and 45,000, or $1,400 and 1,800 per month. In order to elevate the nursing profession and decrease its turnover rate, the Department of Health guided hospitals in improving employee benefits for nurses. For example, new benefits included extended hours for day-care centers, an increased differentials for the night shift, and tuition reimbursement for continued education. Current goals of the Ministry of Education are (a) 15% of the nurses will hold bachelors degrees, (b) 60% will be graduates of junior colleges, and (c) 25% will be vocational school graduates (Chen et al., 1995; Hsiao & Ma, 1996).

According to Chu (1988), different nursing programs produce graduates with different characteristics. For instance, bachelor degree nurses are expected to:

1. Integrate and apply relevant theories and knowledge to the nursing profession.
2. Apply, implement, and improve professional nursing skills.
3. Plan, instruct, and implement teaching activities for an individual or a team.
4. Utilize the communication theories and skills across interdisciplines.

Junior college graduates are expected to:

1. Apply knowledge to the nursing process.
2. Apply and implement professional nursing skills.
3. Follow instruction of teaching activities for an individual or a team.
4. Communicate well with nursing colleagues.

Vocational nursing program graduates are expected to:

1. Apply knowledge of nursing skills.
2. Follow instruction of teaching activities for an individual or a team.
3. Communicate well with nursing colleagues.

Before describing the philosophy of nursing schools in Taiwan, let us interpret the Chinese words for nursing, *hu-li*. According to Liang (1981), the first word, *hu*, means "to protect, to shelter, to harbor, to guard" (p. 488). *Li* means "reason, law, principle, theory, science, to arrange, to administer, to respond" (p. 334).

Due to the trend of Taiwanese students seeking higher education in the United States, more than 50% of the nursing faculty in Tai junior colleges and higher nursing programs are U.S. educated, yet Chinese remains the language of instruction in all schools. Though English textbooks are used in many courses, lectures are in Chinese unless given by a visiting foreign professor. It is not surprising that many of the nursing programs modified the U.S. nursing frameworks, nursing theories, and the nursing models, and adapted them to the curricula in Taiwan.

For example, Roy's Adaptation Model fits into the Chinese cultural and holistic health concept, describing the human being as an adaptive system. "Inputs are mediated by the control process subsystems of cognator and regular coping mechanisms. The system effectors are the adaptive modes. These modes (physiologic, self-concept, role function, and interdependence) are the form in which regulator and cognator subsystems manifest their activity" (Chinn, 1991, p. 187). Chinese health concepts emphasize that prevention is more important than treatment. The human body is considered a whole rather than the sum of its parts, consisting of physical, psychological, and social components. The traditional Chinese health theory includes system concepts and methods. Gold, wood, water, fire, and soil are the five major elements of the human body among which mutual production and destruction exists to form the system in a natural organized way. Moreover, the human race is deemed one of the subsystems of the system-universe and beyond.

Professional Organizations

There are a number of nursing organizations in Taiwan. Those most recognized are discussed below. The NAROC was established in 1961. Its mission is to develop the nursing profession and improve nursing research to elevate the nursing education level. Moreover, NAROC promotes quality of healthcare and collaborates with international nursing organizations. The Nurses' Union of the Republic of China (NUROC) was registered in 1986. Its mission is to organize nurses in order to improve nursing knowledge and position and to ensure the recognition of the nursing profession by the employer and society. The Lamda Beta chapter of the International Honor Society of Nursing, ROC, registered in 1987, strives to improve the international educational information exchange and to consolidate nursing beliefs. Moreover, it promotes the nursing profession and quality of leadership. The Psychiatric Mental Health Nurses Association for the Republic of China (PMHNAROC), and the Long-Term Care Professional Council for the Republic of China (LT-CROC) both were organized in 1992.

Many nursing educators and administrators are actively involved in the international nursing organizations, the most popular being the Sigma Theta Tau International-Honor Society of Nursing. The NAROC is a member of the International Council of Nurses (ICN), and the Department of Health of Taiwan is a member of the World Health Organization (WHO) regional office for the Western Pacific (Shen, 1995; Chu, 1988).

As one of the founding members of the Chinese American Nurses' Association (CANA), I am pleased to announce that CANA was registered in New York State in March 1997. The mission of CANA is to recognize professional Chinese American nurses and to carry out activities on their behalf. In collaboration with other healthcare organizations, its goal is to promote quality healthcare service in the community.

Profiles of Taiwanese Nurses in the United States

Judy Liu, 45-years-old, has been living in the United States nearly 15 years. Currently, she is head nurse in a city hospital. She speaks of her training:

> *"I never encouraged youths to go to the senior vocational school like I did. I had no choice at that time. I had to help my family financially, and, I didn't have a good score on the examination. I was only 15. It was too young to decide or to know what I really wanted for my future. Don't get me wrong, if I don't continue to like nursing, I will not be a nurse for my whole life. The point is that at 15 years' old children are still developing physically and mentally. However, I took the JCEE and used my savings to go back to school for higher education. I had to quit my job in order to be a student at that time. It took a lot of courage to do that. In the vocational school, the faculties were more focused on nursing skill and the teaching style was rigid. Lecture, that's all I can remember. Fifty percent of the time we were in the hospital as student nurses. We also had to go through all of the specialties, (e.g., medicine, surgery, obstetrics, gynecology, psychiatrics, and community health) during each semester. However, in junior college, I learned theories of nursing. We had group projects and presentations. The courses were more exciting than in the vocational school. I felt nursing was nothing until I received a BSN degree in the United States. The RN is more valuable and respected here than in Taiwan. However, I believe that my basic nursing skills are solid because of my vocational education in Taiwan. However, I cannot recall any fun as a teenager because of the long hours."*

Grace Lin, 32-years-old, has been living in the United States for six years and currently is a nurse practitioner (NP) in a city hospital. She speaks of her training in Taiwan and the camaraderie shared among classmates:

> *"I think my five years of junior college in Taiwan are very important to me. I had to spend almost one and a half years as a student nurse in a hospital. But the first three years, we had both an academic high school program and vocational high school program. We did a lot of team papers, group projects, and presentations. Later, I took the JCEE and was accepted by an evening class for my BSN degree, so I didn't need to quit my job. Eight years ago, when I came to the United States for my master's degree, the Taiwanese students' association played an important role during my first two years here. In most of the universities in the United States, as long as they have Taiwanese students, you will find this kind of association to help newcomers quickly adapt to the new environment. You will also find volunteers to help newcomers with rides from the airport, housing, orientation,*

et cetera. One year later, I also became one of the volunteers. Before I came here, I told myself I should make more contact with Americans. Yet, I realized it's so difficult, after more than ten hours of struggling to study in English, I needed to relax by speaking in my native language with Chinese friends. I think that's why the American classmates had the misconception that we wanted to be isolated from others."

THE FUTURE OF TAIWANESE NURSING EDUCATION

Like other developed countries, Taiwan is facing many changes. As the nursing profession moves into the 21st century, we need to have a clear direction and strategic perspectives to face new challenges. First, in order to improve the quality of nursing care, it is important to elevate the nursing education level. One of the short-term goals for the Ministry of Education is to transfer the basic nursing program from vocational school to junior college. Second, the national health insurance system, implemented in 1994, and which provides all Taiwanese citizens with health insurance, continues to aim for cost efficiency for the entire healthcare system. Third, as the aging population in Taiwan continues to increase, nursing will play a significant role especially in the areas of gerontology and chronic diseases, community healthcare, and home healthcare. In response to this trend, nursing leaders should ensure an extended role and function for nurses. Also, nursing curricula should require more science, finance, and administration courses in order to provide professional nurses with critical-thinking skills and creativity to address the needs of society. Finally, a redesign of the nursing education system requires the collaboration of government and nursing schools and organizations. In the future, we expect the Department of Health and Ministry of Education to update policies, implementing systematical continuing education, and to design a framework to produce higher qualified nursing faculty and professional nurses (Shen, 1995).

REFERENCES

Chen, Y. C., Ma, F. C., Lee, Y. Y., Tu, M. S., Wang, W., Yin, T. C., Lu, M. S., Hsiu, N. L., & Lee, H. (1995). *Discussion on professional nursing problems*. Taiwan: Farseeing.

Chu, P. T. (1988). *The history of the nurses' association of the Republic of China*. Taiwan: The Nurses' Association of the Republic of China.

Copper, J. F. (1996). *Taiwan: Nation-state or province?* San Francisco: Westview Press.

Harrell, S., & Huang, C. C. (1994). *Cultural change in postwar Taiwan*. San Francisco: Westview Press.

Hsiao, Y. L., & Ma, F. S. (1996). The correlation among the organizational commitment, organizational retention, and professional retention in clinical nurses. *Nursing Research, 4*(2), p. 137–149.

Hsiung, J. C. (1981). *Contemporary Republic of China: The Taiwan experience 1950–1980*. New York: Praeger.

Liang, S. C. (1985). *Far East concise English-Chinese directory*. Tokyo, Hong Kong, New York: The Far East Book.

Shen, Y. T. (1995). *Introduction of nursing*. Taiwan: Yung-Tai Book.

Smith, D. (1991). *The Confucian continuum: Educational modernization in Taiwan*. New York: Praeger.

CHAPTER THIRTEEN

Traditional Chinese Medicine and Nursing

Shu-Zhen Li, MD

Anli Jiang, MEd

*I*n today's China, nursing has accumulated the wisdom of abundant traditional Chinese medicine and adopted the best of Western science and technology. It signifies an amalgamation of Eastern and Western civilization as well as the integration of traditional characteristics and the spirit of modern science.

BASIC THEORIES OF TRADITIONAL CHINESE NURSING

Traditional Chinese medicine (TCM) has a history of several thousand years. In ancient times, practitioners of TCM provided cures, herbal drug therapy, and long-term care at the same time. In the modern era and after the foundation of the People's Republic of China, many hospitals providing TCM were established. As a result, traditional Chinese nursing (TCN) was given birth and has gradually become a unique science, its characteristics inherited by generations past and future. Actually, the theories of TCM and TCN are almost the same, both stem mainly from practice and have been enriched and expanded through practice. The earliest extant medical classic in China, *Huangdi Neijing (Canon of Medicine),* was compiled between 500 and 300 B.C. and is a summary of the medical experience and theoretical knowledge prior to the Warring period. The book consists of two parts, *Suwen* and *Lingshu,* and describes the basic theories of TCM, such as the concept of the organism as a whole, or *Bian Zheng* (overall analysis of signs and symptoms); *Yin-yang;* the five elements of the human body, channels and collaterals; *qi* (vital energy); and blood. *Huangdi Neijing* also addresses basic knowledge and methods concerning nursing. Following *Neijing,* there appeared quite a number of treatises on traditional medicine in different dynasties. The result is a TCN comprised of many theories with regard to the human body's physiology and pathology, and to the nursing of human health.

The Organism as a Whole

By "organic whole" we mean entirety and unity. TCN attaches great importance to the unity of the human body itself and its relationship with nature, and holds that the body is an organic whole having close and inseparable relations with its external natural surroundings.

Unity Within the Body.   The human body is made up of viscera bowels, tissues, and other organs, each performing its own physiological functions. These different physiological functions comprise the entire life process of the body, determining unity within the body. Therefore, these components are inseparable from each other in structure; they are related, subsidiary and conditional, to each other in physiology, and maintain certain influence upon each other in pathology. The body's mutual relations and influences are centered around the five viscera (heart, liver, spleen, lung, and kidney) and come into effect through channels and collaterals.

Five Viscera	Six Bowels	Five Body	Five Senses
Heart	Small intestine	Vessel	Tongue
Lung	Large intestine	Skin	Nose
Spleen	Stomach	Muscle	Mouth
Liver	Gall bladder	Tendon	Eye
Kidney	Urinary bladder	Bone	Ear
	Excretory systems		
	Urethral orifice		
	and anus		

Unity Between the Human Body and Nature.   Man lives in nature and is influenced directly and indirectly by nature's movements and changes, to which he is bound to make corresponding physiological and pathological responses. For example, as the climate varies throughout the year, normal pulse conditions (pulse rate, rhythm, volume, tension, etc.) likewise vary. Specifically, one's pulse is stringlike in spring, full in summer, floating in autumn, and sunken in winter. These variations provide a basis for doctors to distinguish abnormal pulse conditions during clinical diagnoses. Also seasonal is the occurrence, development, and changes of maladies such as spring's epidemic febrile diseases, summer's sunstrokes, autumn's symptoms of dryness, and winter's cold-stroke syndromes. Of course, people can certainly reduce and even eliminate some seasonal diseases by doing physical exercises, transforming the nature that surrounds them, and taking active measures of prevention. In addition to seasonal variations, traditional Chinese doctors and nurses have observed that certain maladies peak at different times, an alternation in severity whether early morning, late afternoon, day- or nighttime. The monograph titled "Regarding a Day as a Year Consisting of the Four Seasons" (Zhang, 1997) reports:

> *There are various diseases, most of which become milder in the morning, better during the daytime, worse again in the late afternoon and even severer at night. [This is because] in the morning the vital energy of the human body begins to grow stronger, while the pathogenic factor weaker; at midday the vital energy of the human body is predominant and lords it over the pathogenic factors stronger; at midnight, the vital energy of the human body returns to the internal organs, while the pathogenic factors come into leading place. (p. 28)*

More recently, biorhythms have been discovered to affect human pulse conditions and temperature, amount of oxygen consumed and carbon dioxide released, and hormone secretions. This finding may promote round-the-clock exploration of the physiological and pathological changes of the human body.

Based on the theory of the circulation of *qi* characteristics of TCM, the pathogenesis of the human body is often influenced by the periodic climate changes that occur every 12 to 60 years. In recent years, scientists have realized that the law of these periodic changes has something to do with the cycle of sunspots, formed every 11 to 12 years. Their movements cause periodic changes in the radiation of sunlight, interfere with the magnetic field of the earth, and change the climate around the globe, thus exerting a tremendous impact upon the physiology and pathology of the human body.

TCN holds that different geographical surroundings produce different effects on the physiology and pathology of the human body, effects so great as to extend or shorten human lives. *On Conventions of the Five Cirduit Phases* (Zhang, 1997) includes:

People who live in the high areas have a long life, while those who live in the low ones die young. Living areas differ in altitude. A little difference in height causes a little difference in life, while a great difference in height results in a great difference in life. Therefore, physicians have to know the law of nature and geographical conditions. (p. 31)

Modern research shows that mountain areas between 1,500 and 2,000 meters above sea level are ideal geographical locations for a long life, because it is a place where hydrogen anions are concentrated.

Theory of Yin and Yang

Yin and *yang* has historically been considered simply ancient philosophy of China. At first, *Yin* and *yang* denoted whether a place faces the sun— that which is exposed to the sun is *yang,* the other *yin.* For example, the southern side of a mountain is *yang,* while the northern side is *yin.* Subsequently, through long-term living, practice, and observation of every kind of material phenomenon, people have come to realize that *yin* and *yang* exist in all things. Furthermore, their interaction promotes the occurrence, development, and transformation of all things. Consequently, *yin* and *yang* are used as the means of reasoning in analyses of the material world's phenomena. *Lao Zi,* a philosophical work written in ancient China, says, "All things on earth carry *yin* on their backs and hold *yang* in their arms." *Yin* and *yang* have impacted the science of TCM and TCN, prompting the formation and development of these practices' respective theoretical systems.

Prevention

Prevention is to take certain precautions against the occurrence and progression of disease. TCN attaches great importance to prevention. As early as two thousand years ago, the theory of preventive treatment of a disease was put forth in the book *Yellow Emperor's Canon of Internal Medicine.* This theory, in fact, includes two aspects: adopting preventive measures before the onset of disease and taking precautions against the progression of disease.

Taking Preventive Measures.   As previously mentioned, the occurrence of a disease is due to a deficiency of the vital-*qi* and dysfunction of the human body, as well as to the pathological damages to the human body caused by pathogenic factors.

The fluctuation of the vital-*qi* depends primarily on one's constitution. Generally speaking, a man with a strong constitution possesses sufficient vital-*qi* while a constitutionally feeble man has deficient vital-*qi*. Accordingly, it is of crucial importance to strengthen constitution, improving the vital-*qi's* resistance to pathogenic factors. The physical condition of a person is mainly concerned with such aspects as innate characteristics, diet, exercise, and mental state.

One inherits innate characteristics from his or her biological parents. It follows, then, that parents' health status can directly influence the baby's constitution. Many kinds of diseases are associated with genetic factors. In *A Complete Work on Pediatrics,* Chen Fuzheng of the Qin Dynasty wrote, "The majority of the children born by underage parents are weak in constitution." Thereby, late marriage and eugenics should be advocated to ensure children a sound constitution.

To secure one's self with a strong body, he or she should not only understand, but also adapt to the changing patterns of the natural environment. Proper control and arrangement of diet, daily life, work, and rest is essential. According to *Plain Questions,* "One, who knows the ways of health preservation, complies with natural law, adapts himself to the variations in nature, keeps a moderate diet, leads a regular life and shuns overwork, will obtain both physical and mental health which is the promise of longevity of over one hundred years." The book attempts to persuade one not to "drink excessively, indulge himself in sexual measures, act willfully, exhaust all his energies, squander away his essence of life and spirit without any sense of perserving them, follow his aimless inclinations and lead a careless life with no enjoyment of a healthy life."

One's constitution is improved by frequent physical exercise, which strengthens the vital-*qi,* enabling it to combat pathogenic factors as well as reduce or prevent the occurrence of disease. Accelerating the circulation of blood and *qi,* promoting the nimbleness of joints, and keeping the functions and activities of *qi* in good order can be achieved through such physical exercises as the Five-Mimic-Animal boxing created by Doctor Hua Tuo of the Han Dynasty, as well as Taiji boxing, *Baduan Jin, Yijin Jing,* and Chinese *Qigong.* All of these exercises can be done to build up one's constitution and prevent diseases.

A person's mental activities are closely related to the body's physiological and pathological changes. Prevention and treatment of a disease correlate with high spirits and a stable mental state; one should avoid or reduce harmful mental stimulation or overexcitement. According to

Plain Questions, "How can a disease occur if one keeps a serene mind, rejects lust and vain hope, keeps the vital-*qi* in a good condition and maintains a sound mind?"

Prevention via traditional Chinese drugs has been practiced for a long time in China. In recent years, TCM has been making wide use of Chinese medicinal herbs for disease prevention. Satisfactory effects have been obtained in prevention of bacillary dysentery with garlic and portualca oleracea; of virus hepatitis with oriental wormwood, capejasmne, and Chinese dates; and of influenza with isatis leaf and root.

In the sixteenth century, the Chinese invented variolation to prevent smallpox, crowning their country as the world's forerunner in the field of immunology. Modern Chinese doctors have combined traditional medicines with modern immunological techniques to prevent diseases with the result of eradicating such fulminating infections as smallpox and the plague, as well as the effective control of some other communicable diseases.

Pathogenic factors play an important, and sometimes even decisive, role in disease causation. Thus, the preventive treatment of diseases means not only the improvement of constitution and strengthening of the vital-*qi* against pathogenic factors, but also the prevention of the invading pathogenic factors. People should do their utmost to avoid the invasion of pestilence by closely attending to food hygiene. Trauma can be avoided if safety precautions are taken in work and daily life.

Preventing the Progression of a Disease.   It is ideal to prevent disease before it attacks the body. However, once a disease appears, it should be diagnosed and treated as early as possible so as to arrest its progress. Particularly, it is imperative that exopathic diseases be cured at the initial stage in order to check its progression.

Different diseases vary greatly in their progressive patterns. For instance, the miscellaneous diseases caused by internal injury often transform according to the patterns of encroachment and violation of the five elements making up the human body.

The Principle of Nursing

Searching for the Primary Cause of a Disease in Nursing.   In nursing, to search for the primary cause of a disease is to seek the fundamental cause of a disease to ensure proper and appropriate care. This is the basic TCN principle of diagnosis and intervention with regard to analysis of symptoms and signs, cause, nature and location of the illness, and physical condition.

Strengthening the Body's Resistance and Eliminating Pathogenic Factors. Strengthening the vital-*qi* builds the human body's ability for resistance as well as its self-repairing ability to remove pathogens, recovering health. Proven methods include traditional Chinese drugs, acupuncture and moxibustion, and other therapies in combination with proper diet, exercise, and Chinese *qigong.* These techniques can be applied to any kind of deficiency syndrome dominated by the deficiency of the vital-*qi.* Corresponding measures should be adopted in accordance with the disease's specific characteristics. Instances can be found in invigoration *qi* for deficiency of *qi,* enriching blood for lack of blood, and doing both for insufficiency of the two. The same is true of *yin* and *yang* deficiencies. All these are specific approaches to strengthening the body's resistance.

Pathogenic factors may be removed with traditional Chinese drugs or other methods, restoring the vital-*qi* and curing the disease. Corresponding measures should be taken in consideration of the particular kinds and features of pathogens, as well as where they invade.

Regulation of Yin *and* Yang.   The imbalance of *yin* and *yang* turns out to be the fundamental pathogenesis of many diseases. Thus, regulating *yin* and *yang* is essential to maintaining a body's relative balance.

Nursing in Accordance with Seasonal Conditions, Local Conditions, and the Physique of the Individual.   Approaches to nursing must be appropriated according to the various situations, seasons, and regions of care as well as the patient's constitution, sex, and age.

Climatic variations have certain effects on the body's physiology. For instance, in spring and summer, as the weather turns warmer, the *yang-qi* of the body escalates and the muscles and skin relax. For patients with just a bad cold, drastic remedies such as diaphoaetics of ephedra must be used cautiously to avoid inducing too much diaphoresis and thereby impairing *yin.* In autumn and winter, as the weather changes from cool to cold, *yin* becomes increasingly stronger; the muscles close and *yang-qi* is astringent internally. Medicines of cool and cold natures, such as gypsum, mirabilite, and rhubarb should be given with great care.

As with climate, geographical conditions also can affect a person's physiology and pathology.

In reference to the physique of an individual, care plans should suit age, sex, constitution, and lifestyle of the patient.

Older people usually get deficiency syndrome or a combination of both deficiency and excess, since their essence becomes weaker. Such persons should be nursed in a holistic manner with attention to social and spiritual needs, as well as psychological and biological requisites.

Also, the sexes have their own features in physiology and pathology. Strict precautions must be taken in drug administration, especially for women, who are physically characterized by menstruation, leucorrhea, and pregnancy and delivery. Drugs with such features as drastic purgation, removal of blood stasis, and relief of obstruction should be forbidden or administered with great care during the period of pregnancy. Men vary greatly in their constitution and heat index, allowing for one disease to be nursed in several ways. Nurses should understand basic care of infants and children as well as elderly patients.

THEORY OF DIET

Improper diet affects the physiological functions of human beings and reduces resistance to diseases.

It is wise to eat an appropriate amount of food. Excessive hunger and overfeeding both can give rise to diseases. Excessive hunger results in an inadequate intake for the transformation into *qi* and blood, eventually leading to disease. Likewise, overfeeding beyond the normal digestive ability (i.e., hyperphagia) also can give rise to diseases, as well as to indigestion, abdominal distention, and fullness. Because children have weak functions of the spleen and stomach, in addition to a poor sense of proper diet, they are more liable to fall ill. Taken together, an improper diet can cause many kinds of gastrointestinal disease, manifested as diarrhea, abdominal pain, vomiting, purulent and bloody stool, and the like.

Only through an appropriate mixture of food can the human body acquire the various nutrients necessary to sustain life. Herbs and diets have the same source, the same application, the same mechanism. Some foods prevent disease, and some treat disease. Most of the herbs which strengthen the body's constitution and prevent senility are found in good dietary practices. This is the reason why we stress the combination of diet therapy and medical therapy.

BASIC TECHNIQUES OF TRADITIONAL CHINESE NURSING

Nurses of TCN must learn and master time-honored techniques, techniques which are further developed, such as acupuncture, moxibustion, cupping, the *Tuina* and *Qina* methods, medical compress, and so forth. In addition, TCN nurses are instructed in breathing exercises, *Taijiquan, Baduanjin,* animal gestures, and eye exercises. This chapter focuses solely on those TCN techniques used in the clinical setting.

Acupuncture

Acupuncture is a procedure by which disease can be prevented and treated through the proper insertion of needles into pivotal body points and is accompanied by manipulation. Commonly used needles are fili-form, cutaneous, intradermal, and three-edged needle.

Filiform Needle. One of nine needle types used in ancient China, the filiform needle is most widely used. At present, most filiform needles are made of stainless steel. A filiform needle may be divided into five parts (see Figure 13.1).

Tip: Sharp point of needle.
Body: Part between the handle and tip.

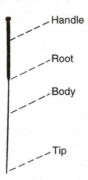

Figure 13.1   Filiform Needle

Root: Connector between body and handle.

Handle: Behind the body, where the hand catches hold of the needle.

Tail: End of handle.

Length and gauge refer to the needle body's dimensions. Filiform needles vary from 1 to 4 inches in length (see Table 13.1).

The needle tip should be as sharp as a pine needle and the body should be round and smooth, flexible and resilient. Needles should be carefully stored to avoid damage, and tips should be preserved with special care by observing the following instructions:

Unused needles should be stored in a box with layers of gauze or in a tube with dry cotton balls placed at both ends to protect the tip. When sterilizing with boiling water, needles should be bound steadily by gauze to prevent the tip from hitting against the autoclave wall. Needle insertion should be neither too forceful nor too fast to prevent it from bending. If the needle tip touches bone, the needle should be withdrawn slightly to avoid bending.

Needling Practice.   It is difficult to insert the filiform needle into the skin as it is. An appropriate finger force guarantees minimum pain and maximum therapeutic effect. The training of fingers may start with a short and thick filiform needle, progressing to a finer and longer instrument before clinical application.

Practice with sheets of paper. Fold fine and soft tissue into a small packet about 5 × 8 cm in size and 1 cm in thickness. Bind the packet with gauze thread. Hold the paper packet in the left hand and the needle in the right, inserting the needle into the packet and rotating it clockwise and counterclockwise (see Figure 13.2 on the following page). At the beginning, if you feel the needle is stuck or difficult to rotate, slow your efforts and continue the exercise. As your finger force grows stronger, the thickness of the paper may be increased.

One also may practice with a cotton cushion. Make a cotton cushion about 5 to 6 cm in diameter with gauze. Hold the cushion with the left hand and needle with the right. Insert the needle into the cushion and practice rotating, lifting, and thrusting procedures (see Figure 13.3 on the following page). Practice basic manipulation techniques according to

Table 13.1   Gauge of Filiform Needle

No.	26	28	30	32	34
Diameter (cm)	0.45	0.38	0.32	0.26	0.22

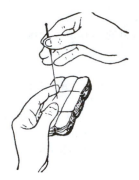

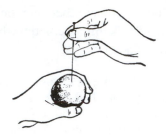

Figure 13.3   Practicing Needling on
Cotton Cushion

Figure 13.2   Practicing Needling on
Folded Paper

the required posture during acupuncture and the reinforcing and reducing approach.

Equipment and Procedure.   Needles should be thoroughly inspected and sanitized. Before performing acupuncture, gather needles of various sizes, trays, forceps, moxe wool, jars, sterilized cotton balls, and 75% alcohol or 1.5% iodine. Carefully inspect and prepare tincture before use.

When sterilizing needles in an autoclave, set atmospheric pressure at 1.5 and $1.2cm^2$ (per square centimeter) for 30 minutes. Of course, the easy and effective method is to boil needles in water for 15 to 20 minutes, which requires no special equipment. But if medical sterilization is pursued, soak the needles in 75% alcohol 30 to 60 minutes. Take them out of the solution and wipe off the liquid with a piece of sterilized dry cloth. One should be careful with instruments made of glass and those with less heat resistance, soaking them in bromogeramin solution (1:1000) for 1 to 2 hours.

Appropriate posturing of the patient is essential to locate pivotal points and manipulate for acupuncture. Generally, the nurse must be able to work without hindrance, and the patient must be relaxed. Postures adopted in the clinic setting are as follows:

Supine: Suitable for the points on the head and face, chest and abdominal region, the medial side of the upper limbs, the anterior side of the lower limbs, and the hands and feet (see Figure 13.4).

Prone: Suitable for the points on the posterior of head, neck, back, lumbar, and buttock regions, and the posterior part of the lower limbs (see Figure 13.5).

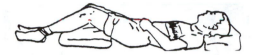

Figure 13.4   Supine Posture

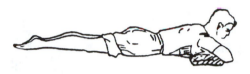

Figure 13.5   Prone Posture

Lateral Recumbent: Suitable for the points on the hind head, neck, and back (see Figure 13.6).

Sitting.

Sitting Erect with Elbows Flexed on Table: Suitable for the points on the forehead, face, neck, and upper portion of the chest (see Figure 13.7 on the following page).

Sitting in Flexion: Suitable for the points on the head, neck, and back (see Figure 13.8 on the following page).

Before acupuncture treatment, the nurses should clean their hands and fingers with soap and water or with an alcohol swab.

The acupuncture area also must be disinfected. The area on the body surface selected for needling should be sterilized with a 75% alcohol cotton ball (or first with 2.5% tincture of iodine, removed by 75% alcohol). Avoid polluting the disinfected area by keeping soiled articles away from the patient's skin.

The needle should be inserted coordinately with both hands. The posture for insertion should be correct so that the manipulation will be smooth. Generally, the needle should be held with the right hand, known

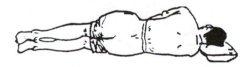

Figure 13.6   Lateral Recumbent

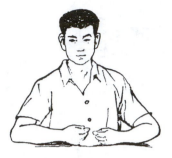

Figure 13.7   Sitting Erect with
Elbows Flexed on Table

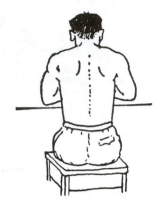

Figure 13.8   Sitting in Flexion

as the puncturing hand; the left hand, known as the pressing hand, presses the area or supports the needle body. The function of the puncturing hand is to hold the needle and perform manipulation; the other hand's function is to fix upon the location of a point and aid needle insertion. Commonly used insertions are as follows:

> Finger Press Insertion: Press on the acupuncture point with nail of the thumb or index finger, or the middle finger on the left hand. Hold the needle with the right hand, keeping the tip close against the border of the giding, and then insert the needle into the skin (see Figure 13.9). This method is suitable for puncturing with short needles.

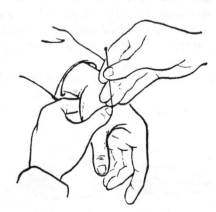

Figure 13.9   Finger Press Insertion

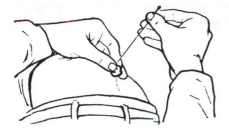

Figure 13.10   Pinch Needle Method

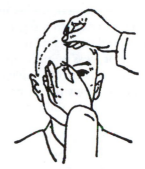

Figure 13.11   Pinch Skin Method

Pinch Needle Method: Hold the dried sterilized cotton ball around the needle tip with the thumb and index fingers of the left hand. Fix the needle tip directly over the selected point, holding its handle with the right hand. Then, while the right hand presses the needle downward, the thumb and index fingers of the left hand insert the tip into the skin (see Figure 13.10). This method is suitable for puncturing with long needles.

Pinch Skin Method: Pinch up the skin around the puncture point with the thumb and index fingers of the left hand, and hold the needle with the right hand. Insert the needle into the pinched skin (see Figure 13.11). This method is suitable for puncturing points on areas where muscles and skin are thin.

Tight Skin Method: Put the thumb and index fingers or index and middle fingers on the skin where the point is located, and separate the two fingers and stretch. Insert the needle (see Figure 13.12). This method is suitable for puncturing points on areas where skin is loose.

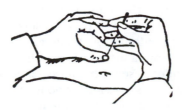

Figure 13.12   Tight Skin Method

The needle methods mentioned are flexible and may be adopted according to the anatomic feature of the area where the point is located and the required depth and manipulation.

In the process of insertion, angle and depth are especially important in acupuncture. Correct angle and depth help to induce the needling sensation, bring about the desired therapeutic results, and guarantee patient safety. Generally, there are three kinds of angle insertion:

Perpendicular: The needle is inserted perpendicularly, forming a 90° angle with the skin's surface. Most points on the body can be punctured in this way.

Oblique: The needle is inserted obliquely to form an approximate angle of 45° with the skin surface. This method is used for points in which deep insertion is not advisable or to avoid puncturing blood vessels and scarring.

Horizontal (also known as subcutaneous or transverse insertion): The needle is inserted transversely to form an angle of 15° to 25° with the skin. This method is suitable for points on the thin skin or muscle and penetrated points.

Depth of needle insertion depends on the pathological condition and location of points; different constitutions and body types provide for different needling sensations; therefore, the depth of insertion must be fully considered according to the body's concrete condition, location of points, and patient characteristics. Only by doing so can better therapeutic results be obtained.

Needling manipulation, also known as needling transmission, refers to various manipulations of acupuncture to induce needling sensation after insertion. During this needling sensation, the patient may experience soreness, numbness, distention, or heaviness around the point. Sometimes the patient may feel warmth, itching, or pain. A feeling of electric shock or of crawling ants is also possible. At the same time, the nurse may feel a tenseness and should drag the sensation around the needle.

There are many factors influencing the arrival of *qi,* the main ones of which are related to constitution of patient, severity of illness, location of points, and needling manipulation. Generally speaking, patients with abundant channel *qi,* or *qi* and blood, may have a rapidly developed needling sensation, while those with excess *yin* and deficient *yang* may experience a slow needling sensation or none. Accurate location of the points makes needling sensation occur rapidly, but in the case of inaccurate location, it is not easy for needling sensation to come. Proper needling manipulations, such as prolonged retaining and pressing of the skin along the channel's course, may promote the movement of the channel *qi* to reach the point.

Manipulation techniques can be divided into two types: fundamental and auxiliary. They may be used either alone or in combination according to the concrete conditions of the patient clinically.

Fundamental manipulation techniques refer to basic actions in acupuncture. The two commonly used techniques follow:

Lifting and Thrusting: This is a method by which the needle body is perpendicularly lifted then thrusted into the point. Thrusting means to insert the needle from the superficial layer to the deep layer; then on the contrary, to withdraw the needle from the deep layer to the superficial layer.

Twirling or Rotating: This refers to the manipulation by which the needle body is twirled or rotated forward and backward until the needle reaches its desired depth. Manipulation is done by the thumb, middle, and index fingers of the right hand, which holds the needle body.

Auxiliary manipulations include pressing, plucking, scraping, shaking, and flying:

Pressing: Slightly press the skin up and down along the course of the channel with the fingers. This is a method of promoting *qi* by which the circulation of *qi* and blood is pushed and the channel *qi* is promoted to reach the diseased part of the body.

Plucking: In the process of retaining, pluck the needle handle slightly with the finger, causing it to tremble and strengthen the stimulation to obtain *qi*.

Scraping: After the needle is inserted to a certain depth, scrape the handle with the nail of the thumb, index, or middle finger of the right hand upward. Scraping is a method of promoting *qi*. It is used to spread the needling sensation.

Shaking: After the needle is inserted to a certain depth, shake the needle with the handle. Shaking is a method of conducting the *qi* flow and needle sensation in a certain direction.

Flying: After the needle is inserted to a certain depth, twirl the needle, allowing your thumb and index fingers to "fly." The two fingers separate just like a flying bird spreading its wings. This method can induce the spread of the channel *qi* and make the therapeutic result better.

Once the needle is inserted into a point, it is retained, or kept in place. The purpose of retaining is to strengthen the needling sensation and to facilitate manipulation of the needle. In general, the needle is retained for 10 to 20 minutes; but for special cases, retaining time may be appropriately prolonged. Meanwhile, manipulations are given to the patient at intervals, strengthening the therapeutic effects. For instance, with a dull needling sensation, retaining the needle serves as a method to wait for *qi* to arise.

After manipulating or retaining the needle, withdraw it from the skin. Press the skin around the point with the thumb and index finger of the left hand, gently rotating the needle and lifting it slowly to the subcutaneous level. Then withdraw the needle quickly and press the punctured point with an alcohol cotton ball to prevent bleeding.

Management of Possible Accidents.   Fainting is due to improper positioning, nervous tension, delicate constitution, and forceful manipulation. The manifestations are sudden dizziness, nausea and vomiting, pallor, palpitation, shortness of breath, drop in blood pressure, cold extremities, and thin and rapid or deep-sited pulse. In severe cases, there may be loss of consciousness, a sudden fall, cyanosis of lips and fingernails, and fecal and urinary incontinence. In case of fainting, stop needle insertion immediately and withdraw those needles already in effect. Comfort the patient and offer warm water. The symptoms will disappear after a short rest. In severe cases, press hard with the fingernail or needle *ZenZhong, Suliao,* and *Neiguan,* and apply moxibustion to *baihui* and *Guanyuan* to wake the patient. If the patient does not respond to the above measures, other emergency measures should be taken.

Stuck needles account for difficult or impossible manipulations. If the needle is stuck, manage it according to its cause. If it is due to a local muscle spasm, ask the patient to relax, leave the needle in place for a while, then withdraw it by rotating or massaging the skin near the insertion point. If the stuck needle is caused by excessive rotation in one direction, the condition will be overcome when the needle is twirled in the opposite direction, loosening bound muscle fibers. After the condition is released, withdraw the needle.

Bent needles may result from unskilled or too forceful manipulation, the needle's striking hard tissue, a change of the patient's posture after insertion, collision of the needle's handle with some external force, and improper management of a stuck needle. When the needle is bent slightly, rotating must not be applied. If the needle is bent severely, it may be withdrawn by following the bend's course. In case the bent needle is caused by a change in the patient's position, remove the needle.

Broken needles arise from too strong manipulations of the needle after insertion—strong muscle spasms, and sudden movements of the patient after the needle is in place. When a needle breaks, nurses must keep calm and ask patients not to move in order to prevent the broken needle from going deeper into the body. If the broken part protrudes from the skin, remove it with forceps; if it is completely under the skin, surgical operation is required.

Subcutaneous bleeding may cause a mild hematoma. This will disappear by itself, but if local swelling and pain are severe, the hematoma is large and affects the motor functions. First, apply a cold compress to the area of the hematoma to stop bleeding; then apply a warm compress, pressing or lightly massaging to disperse and absorb the local stases of blood.

The pleura and lung are sometimes injured when acupuncture is applied to points above the superclavicular fossa, or the suprasternal notch; both sides of the eleventh thoracic vertebra; points above the eighth intercostal space on the middle auxillary line; and above the sixth intercostal space on the midclavicular line. When this occurs, air enters the thoracic cavity, causing pneumothorax. The patient may suddenly feel chest oppression and pain, shortness of breath, and even dyspnea. Also, there may be symptoms of shock, such as cyanosis, sweating, and a drop in blood pressure. Examination may reveal a wider intercostal space of the disease. A hyperresonance may be gotten on thoracic percussin. The vesicular respiratory sound becomes weak or disappears. The trachea is displaced to the healthy side. Further diagnosis of the condition is confirmed by chest X-rays. Once pneumothorax takes place, ask the patient to rest in a half cumbent posture. Mild cases can be managed according to symptoms and signs. If the patient has a cough, antitussive and antibiotics, or antipholgistics, are to be given. For severe cases, emergency measures such as sacking out air by thoracentesis, oxygen inhalation, anti-shock therapy, and so forth, should be taken.

Moxibustion

Moxibustion is an external method of preventing and treating diseases by ignition of moxa to stimulate the body's pressure points. The material mainly used is moxa wool, which is made of moka leaves dried, grounded, and sieved. The leaves are fragrant and easily ignited. Used for several thousand years by acupuncturists and nurses, moxa leaves warm channels and expel cold to induce smooth flow of *qi* and blood, subdue swelling, and disperse accumulation of targeted pathogen(s). There are many types of moxibustion, and the technique utilizes moxa cones and sticks, and warming needles.

Moxa cones are made from kneaded and shaped moxa wool (see Figure 13.13). Cones vary in size, some as big as a grain of wheat. During treatment with moxibustion, whether direct or indirect, the moxa cone when used at a point is called one unit, or one *Zhuang*.

When direct moxibustion, a moxa cone is placed directly on the skin and ignited (see Figure 13.14), and is also known as open moxibustion. This technique is divided into nonscarring and scarring moxibustion, according to different degrees of burnt skin.

Nonscarring moxibustion, also known as nonfestering moxibustion, involves a moxa cone of proper size placed directly on a point and ignited until the local skin becomes ruddy. (There should be no scar formation after moxibustion.) Prior to application, apply a small amount of Vaseline to the area around the point to increase adhesion of the moxa cone to the skin. Place a moxa cone on the point and ignite. When three-fifths to three-fourths of the moxa cone is burnt or if the patient feels pain, remove the cone and replace it with another one.

Like the nonscarring method, scarring moxibustion, also known as festering moxibustion, involves putting a moxa cone directly on a point and igniting it. But this method is characterized by a local blister, festering, and scarred skin around the point after healing. Prior to moxibustion, apply garlic juice to the point. Once the moxa cone burns completely, remove the ash and repeat the procedure according to the required units of moxa cones. Reapply garlic juice to the point after each unit of moxa cone is used. If the patient feels burning pain, the nurse may pat gently on the skin around the point to alleviate the pain. Festering appears and

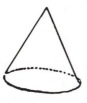

Figure 13.13	Moxa Cone

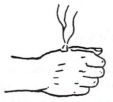

Figure 13.14	Direct Moxibustion

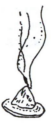

Figure 13.15   Moxibustion with Ginger

post-moxibustion sores form a week after moxibustion. After approximately 45 days, the moxibustion sore may heal, leaving a scar on the skin.

Indirect moxibustion is performed by igniting the moxa cone insulated from the skin by a pad of some substance. This practice is classified according to the various medical substances used for insulation; for example, moxibustion with ginger, garlic, or salt (see Figure 13.15).

To perform moxibustion with moxa sticks, roll moxa wool into the shape of a cylinder, using paper. Ignite one end and put it over the selected point of the body. Moxibustion with moxa is easy to manipulate, the therapeutic effect is good, and the method is easily accepted by patients.

Manipulation and Precautions.   Moxibustion is generally applied to upper body parts first and then to lower body parts. Treat the back first, the abdominal region second, then the head and four extremities. Apply to *yang* channels first, then to *yin* channels. Use lesser units, gradually increasing the number during treatment.

The volume for moxibustion, including the size of the moxa cone or duration of the moxa stick application, should parallel the patient's pathological conditions, general constitution, age, and the site where moxibustion is applied. Generally, three to five units of moxa cones are used for each point, twenty minutes for the application of moxa sticks.

Scarring moxibustion should not be applied to the face, pericardia region, area of the large blood vessels, and regions of the muscles and tendons. Also, it is not advised for the abdominal region of men and women and lumbosacral region of pregnant women.

For patients with coma, numbness of the extremities, or dysesthesia, excessive dosage of moxibustion is not advisable.

Sometimes, blisters result on the skin after moxibustion. Small blisters can heal themselves, but large blisters should be punctured with a sterilized needle and drained, then dressed with anticeptic gauze.

After scarring moxibustion, the patient should not participate in strenuous physical labor and must keep the local skin clean to avoid infection during suppuration of the post-moxibustion sore. If the sore does become infected, apply antiphlogistic plaster to it.

Cupping Therapy

Cupping therapy is mainly used to treat arthralgia syndrome due to wind-dampness, various nervous paralysis, and diseases in the gastrointestinal and lung regions. The procedure involves a jar attached to the skin's surface to cause local congestion through removal of the air in the jar. This is created by introducing heat in the form of an ignited material. This method has the function of warming and promoting the free flow of *qi* and blood in channels, diminishing swellings and pains, and dispelling cold and dampness. Commonly used jars include the following:

> Bamboo Jar: Cut down a section of bamboo 3 to 5 cm in diameter and 6 to 8 or 8 to 10 cm in length, forming a pipe. One thick end is used as the middle part of the jar. The rim of the jar should be made smooth by a piece of sand paper (see Figure 13.16). The bamboo jar is light, economical and uneasy to break, but easy to crack with dryness.
>
> Pottery Jar: Made of pottery clay by means of baking, the jar is shaped as a waist drum, its mouth smooth, with both ends smaller and the middle part extended slightly. The pottery jar is characterized by a big force of suction, but easy to break.
>
> Glass Cup: The mouth of the cup is smooth and small, but the body is large, and the rim of the mouth everted externally. The cup is

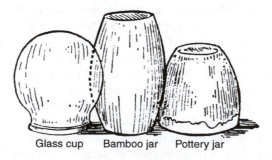

Glass cup   Bamboo jar   Pottery jar

Figure 13.16   Commonly Used Jars in Cupping Therapy

transparent, so congestion of the local skin can be seen to control the time of treatment. The glass cups are easy to break.

Manipulation and Precautions.   Place an ignited alcohol cotton ball or a piece of ignited paper into the cup, then rapidly place the mouth of the cup firmly against the selected site. Clamp an ignited alcohol cotton ball with forceps, move it around the inner wall of the cup and immediately put it on the selected site.

Generally, the cup is sucked for 10 minutes. When the local skin becomes congested with violet-colored blood stasis formation, the cup is withdrawn. On withdrawing the cup, hold it with the right hand and press the skin around the rim of the cup with thumb and index finger of the left hand to let in air, then remove the cup.

It is not advisable to apply cupping to the patient with skin ulcers, high fever and convulsions, or skin allergies.

Uneven sites around joints and the areas with very loose skin are not selected for cupping.

The Three-Edged Needle

The three-edged needle, once known as the ensiform needle, is shaped by a thick and round handle, triangular body, and sharp tip. Generally, it is used to cause bleeding by superficial pricking of the blood vessel. Specifically, the technique is used to promote the smooth flow of *qi* and blood in the body's channels. It is advisable to treat blockage of the channels, blood stasis, pathogenic excess, and blockage of both *yin-qi* and *yang-qi*.

Manipulation and Precautions.   Spot prickings is a method used to treat fever, sore throat, heat stroke, apoplexy, and the like. During the operation, pinch the selected area tightly with the thumb, index, and middle fingers of the left hand; hold the needle with the right hand, pricking swiftly at the area. Withdraw the needle immediately, then squeeze and press the local area for blood letting.

Clumpy pricking is indicated in carbuncles, arthralgia syndrome, and crysiplas. Apply the routine sterilization around a reddened swelling; prick around the lesion several times with a three-edged needle, then squeeze and press the swelling.

Pricking is suitable for the hands, chest, back, and face, and for areas with thin muscles. During the operation, point to the local reactive spot and pinch up the muscle around it with the three-edged needle held in the right hand to encourage bleeding.

Strict sterilization must be applied to the pricked area. The operation should be slight, superficial, and quick. Bleeding should not be excessive. Avoid injuring deep large arteries. Pricking should not be applied to those with a weak constitution or anemia, pregnant women, parturixents, and those susceptible to bleeding.

REFERENCES

Cheng, X. (1987). *Chinese acupuncture and moxibustion*. Publishing House of Foreign Language.

Historical Publications: *Huangdi's Internal Classic; Miraculous Pivot; Plain Questions; Synopsis of Prescription from the Golden Chamber.*

Wu, X. (1991). *Traditional Chinese nursing*. Publishing House of Shanghai University of Traditional Chinese Medicine.

Zhang, E. (1997). *Basic theory of traditional Chinese medicine (1) and (2)*. Publishing House of Shanghai University of Traditional Chinese Medicine.

Zhang, E. (1997). *Chinese acupuncture and moxibustion*. Publishing House of Shanghai University of Traditional Chinese Medicine.

Index

AAPI, *see* Asian American Pacific Islander (AAPI), health promotion interventions for

Aborigines, in Taiwan, 188

Abortion, induced (Korean women), 52–53

Acupuncture, 204–213
  equipment and procedure, 206–212
  filiform needle, 204–205
  management of possible accidents, 212–213
  needling practice, 205–206

Acute/chronic problems, Korean women, 50–51

Aging:
  Chinese view of (*Xi Young Hong*), 26, 27
  phenomenon of, 26–27

AIDS, *see* HIV/AIDS

Alcohol use, 21
  and Korean women, 47–48
  and risk for AIDS, 91

Amor propio, 69

APICHA (Asian and Pacific Islander Coalition for HIV/AIDS), 94

APITEN (Asian Pacific Islander Tobacco Education Network), 12

APPEAL (Asian Pacific Partners for Empowerment and Leadership), 12

Arbularyos, 71

Asian, and/or Asian American:
  Asian Indian, *see* Indians, Asian
  Chinese, *see* China/Chinese/Chinese-Americans; Chinese American elderly immigrants ("King City"/New York study); Chinese American women, older, qualitative study of health practice in; Chinese nursing, traditional (TCN)
  Filipino, *see* Filipino/Filipino-Americans
  Japanese, *see* Japan/Japanese Americans; Japan: public health and medical care, changes/strategies
  Korean, *see* Korea/Koreans
  largest populations, 5
  subgroups, 4, 12, 87–88
  Taiwanese, *see* Taiwan/Taiwanese

Asian American Pacific Islander (AAPI), health promotion interventions for, 3–15
  and cancer, 5–6
  and cardiovascular disease (CVD), 4–5
  conclusion, 12–13

219